Mindful Motherhood

Guided Meditations and Real Conversation for
Busy Mamas

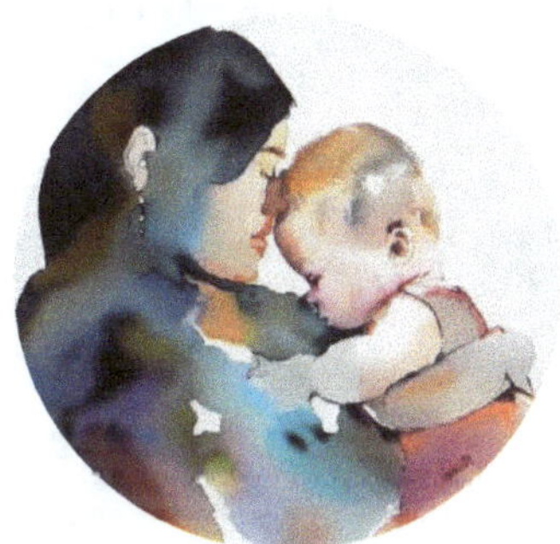

Written by

Dr. Hannah M. Mecaskey Conley, LICSW, LABA

Illustrations Developed with AI from OpenArt.ai

COPYRIGHT INFORMATION

contents

contents

Preface

EMBRACING IMPERFECTION: A MOTHER'S JOURNEY

Preface: Embracing Imperfection - A Mother's Journey

Dear Reader,

As you embark on this journey through the pages of this book, I want to extend a warm welcome and offer a heartfelt disclaimer. Whether you are reading this as an individual or part of group, the resources you're about to explore were crafted from one mother's perspective—one who has worn many hats throughout her life. I am a therapist, a friend, a colleague to other mothers, but above all, a mother myself.

These pages are not the product of an infallible expert dispensing wisdom from a pedestal of perfection. Instead, they are born from the depths of my own journey—a journey through the joys and trials of motherhood. They are the result of countless conversations with mothers from all walks of life, sharing their hopes, their struggles, and their victories.

I've walked alongside mothers in therapy sessions, in coffee shops, and in the quiet corners of our hearts. I've seen the courage it takes to navigate the complex terrain of motherhood, to wrestle with doubts, to celebrate small wins, and to face moments of vulnerability head-on.

This book is not a one-size-fits-all guide; rather, they are an offering from a fellow traveler on this beautiful, messy, and often unpredictable journey. My perspective is shaped by my own experiences, my work as a therapist, and the profound connections I've made with other mothers.

From a desire to support hope, healing, and self-acceptance, I've woven together meditations, reflections, and affirmations to accompany you on your path. They are not solutions to all of life's challenges, but rather tools to help you navigate them with grace and resilience.

In these pages, you will find chapters that explore the intricate dance of motherhood, from centering after a long day to embracing imperfection. They are an invitation to pause, reflect, and connect with your own journey.

But please remember, these resources are not a substitute for professional advice or guidance. If you find yourself grappling with complex emotions or facing challenges that seem insurmountable, I encourage you to seek support from a therapist or counselor who can provide the personalized care you deserve.

As you read, I invite you to embrace the imperfection within these pages. They are offered with the knowledge that we are all works in progress, that motherhood is a journey filled with both light and shadow, and that it's through our shared experiences and compassionate connections that we find our way.

So, dear reader, may these resources be a source of comfort, inspiration, and self-acceptance on your unique journey through motherhood. Know that you are not alone, that your imperfections are part of what makes you beautifully human, and that there is hope and healing to be found in every step.

With warmth and understanding,

CHAPTER 01

Chapter 1: Centering After a Long Day

After a long day of juggling the demands of your career and the responsibilities of motherhood, it's entirely normal to feel torn. On one hand, you have a deep love for your work, a sense of pride in your accomplishments, and the knowledge that your professional pursuits contribute to your family's well-being. On the other hand, there's that maternal ache in your heart, a longing to be with your children, to hold them close, and to be present for every moment of their growth.

This internal tug-of-war can be emotionally challenging. You might question if you're giving enough to either role or if you're striking the right balance. It's essential to recognize that these feelings are a testament to the depth of your love for both your career and your children.

Take a moment to reflect on the following:

1. **You Are Not Alone:** Many working mothers experience these conflicting emotions. It's a shared journey, and you are not alone in this struggle.
2. **The Power of Presence:** While you may not always be physically present with your children, remember that your love transcends physical boundaries. When you are with

them, make those moments count by being fully present and engaged.

3. **Prioritizing Self-Care:** It's crucial to care for yourself, both professionally and personally. By nurturing your own well-being, you become better equipped to fulfill your roles effectively.

4. **Celebrate Achievements:** Acknowledge and celebrate your achievements at work. Your success is not only a source of pride but also an inspiration for your children, showing them the importance of pursuing their dreams.

5. **Forgiveness and Compassion:** Be gentle with yourself. There will be days when you excel at both your career and motherhood, and days when you may feel stretched. Embrace imperfection and practice self-compassion.

Remember, you are a remarkable woman, capable of achieving greatness in your career and providing boundless love as a mother.

The balancing act may be challenging, but it's in these moments of reflection that you find the strength to navigate the beautiful, complex journey of being a working mother. Your love for your children and your dedication to your career *can* coexist harmoniously in your life.

Meditation: Finding Your Inner Calm

Find a comfortable and quiet space where you won't be disturbed. Sit or lie down, whichever feels best for you.

Close your eyes, take a deep breath in, and exhale slowly.

Feel any tension in your body start to melt away with each breath.

Imagine a warm, soothing light surrounding you, wrapping you in a cocoon of calm and tranquility. This light represents your inner calm.

Visualize the events of your busy day like leaves floating on a gentle stream.

Each leaf represents a task, a worry, or a stressor.

Watch them float away, leaving you feeling lighter and freer.

Now, turn your attention inward. Focus on your breath, the rise, and fall of your chest or abdomen.

Feel the rhythm of your breath, like the gentle waves of the ocean.

As you breathe, repeat the following words in your mind:

"I am a calm and capable mother, no matter what the day brings."
Visualize yourself handling challenges with grace and ease.
Picture yourself as the calm center of your family, radiating peace and love.
Take a few more deep breaths, inhaling positivity and exhaling any remaining tension or doubts.
When you're ready, slowly open your eyes, returning to the present moment, carrying this sense of inner calm with you.

Affirmation

"I am a calm and capable mother, no matter what the day brings."

Repeat this affirmation whenever you need to re-center and remind yourself of your inner strength.

You are a capable and loving mother who can navigate any challenges that come your way with grace and calmness

A Personal Note on Centering
After a Long Day

As I reflect on the challenges and triumphs of this chapter, I'm reminded of just how important it is to find a moment of centering after a long day. It's a time to reconnect with ourselves, our partners, and our families, but it's not always easy in a world filled with distractions.

At the end of a busy day, when work commitments, household chores, and the demands of parenting have tugged at us from every direction, the need to center ourselves becomes even more critical. It's a time to pause, take a deep breath, and remind ourselves of the importance of presence.

But let's be honest—centering is not always a seamless process. There are moments when it feels like the world is pulling us in a hundred different directions, and finding that inner calm can be a challenge. The notifications on our phones keep pinging, the to-do list keeps growing, and the worries of the day can linger.

Yet, it's precisely in those challenging moments that centering becomes most vital. It's a reminder that we have the power to reclaim our focus, to disconnect from the noise, and to be fully present with ourselves and our loved ones.

So, as we embark on this journey of exploring the art of centering after a long day, let's acknowledge the difficulties that may arise and find solace in the fact that we are not alone in this struggle. We're all learning and growing, one centering moment at a time.

In the chapters ahead, we'll delve deeper into the practices that can help us achieve that much-needed sense of calm and connection.

Together, we'll navigate the challenges of Millennial motherhood and find our way back to a place of centering, where love, presence, and inner peace prevail.

CHAPTER
02

Chapter 2: Release Stress and Tension

As a busy working mother, it's natural to carry the weight of the day's stress and worries with you. But in order to be truly present for your children, it's important to let go of these tensions and embrace peace in this moment.

In the journey of motherhood, particularly for those who are also dedicated to their careers, it's not uncommon to feel like you're constantly being pulled in multiple directions. The daily juggle between professional responsibilities, personal ambitions, and the nurturing role of motherhood can create a whirlwind of stress and tension.

As you've sat down to release the day's stress and tension, you may have recognized the multitude of roles you play: the capable professional, the loving mother, the partner, the friend, and so many more. Each role carries its own set of expectations and demands, tugging at your time and energy.

As we practiced in the previous chapter's meditation, we must let go of the tensions and stressors that pull at us each day when transitioning between our professional and maternal roles. In doing so, we release what no longer serves us and making room for the peace and presence we deserve.

Here are some thoughts to ponder:

1. **Balancing Act:** You are a remarkable woman who wears many hats. Remember that it's not about being perfect in each role every day but finding balance over time.
2. **Prioritizing Presence:** Being present with your children doesn't mean being physically there all the time. It's about making the moments you have count, about quality over quantity.
3. **Self-Care:** Releasing stress is an act of self-care. By taking care of yourself, you become better equipped to care for others. It's not selfish; it's essential.
4. **Embracing Imperfection:** Perfection is an unattainable goal. Embrace your imperfections, knowing that it's okay to ask for help and take breaks when needed.
5. **Setting Boundaries:** Consider setting boundaries to protect your precious time and energy. It's a powerful tool for maintaining balance.
6. **Celebrate Achievements:** Celebrate your successes, both big and small. Acknowledge your ability to manage and excel in your various roles.

As you continue your journey, keep in mind that you are not alone in this experience. Countless mothers have navigated these waters before you and will do so after you. By finding moments to release stress and tension and embracing peace in the present, you empower yourself to be the loving and capable mother your children need, while also nurturing your own well-being. It's a journey of self-discovery, resilience, and, above all, love

Meditation: Letting Go of the Day's Stress

Find a comfortable and quiet space where you can sit or lie down. Close your eyes gently, and take a few deep breaths in and out to settle into this moment.

Imagine yourself at the end of a busy workday.

See your workplace, the tasks you've accomplished, and the people you've interacted with.

These are the priorities and responsibilities you've carried throughout the day.

As you sit with these images, acknowledge the dedication and effort you've put into your work.

Recognize that you've done your best, and now it's time to shift your focus to what truly matters: your family.

In your mind, gather all the tasks, emails, and to-dos from your workday.

Imagine placing them aside, on as safe place in your workspace.

Your work concerns are now safe, and your priorities will be held for you until tomorrow. Release them.

As you release each work-related item from your conscious thoughts, feel a sense of relief and lightness.

Your work responsibilities are safe and secure here.

Visualize a transitional space, like a threshold, between your work life and your family life. Picture this space as a beautiful garden where the sun is setting, casting a warm, golden glow.

Now, visualize your family waiting for you just beyond the garden.

See their smiling faces, filled with love and anticipation for your presence.

As you step through the threshold from work to family, imagine that you're shedding a heavy cloak of stress and responsibility.

Feel it slide off your shoulders and fall away.

With your workday behind you, take a deep breath and become fully aware of the here and now. Listen to the sounds of your family members, their laughter, and the comforting noises of your home.

Feel the solid ground beneath you, supporting you as you transition.

Sense the peace and tranquility of this moment as you immerse yourself in your family's warm embrace.

As you stand in the garden of transition, check-in with yourself to take a temperature internally.

Remember to pause and honor your own needs, as self-care is a vital part of maintaining balance and well-being.

Take a few moments to savor this transition. When you're ready, open your eyes, carrying with you the intention to be fully present with your family and to nurture yourself with self-care.

You have the capacity to gracefully transition from work to family life, embracing each moment with love and intention.

The cares of your career are not so fragile, nor are they so important, that they need to flood your day beyond the work space.

Affirmation

"I release work care and embrace the remainder of my moments with family!"

Repeat this affirmation as you continue to breathe deeply and visualize the stress leaving your body.

With each breath, you let go a little more, making space for the joy and presence you wish to share with your children.

When you're ready, slowly open your eyes, carrying this newfound sense of peace and presence into your interactions with your loved ones.

By releasing the day's stress and embracing peace in the present moment, you empower yourself to be fully present and engaged with your children, creating cherished moments together

CHAPTER 03

Chapter 3: Mindful Evening Routines

In the hustle and bustle of daily life, it's easy to rush through our evening routines without truly being present. But by embracing mindful moments, you can nurture a sense of presence and connection with your family.

One of the most powerful lessons I've learned is the importance of creating screen-free zones and designated times for family in the evening. In our fast-paced world, screens can easily take over our lives, leaving little room for meaningful connections with our loved ones.

By setting boundaries around screen time, we can reclaim the space of the home for quality family interactions. Opening ourselves to the beauty of unplugged moments in the evening. When we put away our devices and focus on being present with our family members, we create a space for genuine conversations, shared laughter, and deeper connections. These moments of presence are priceless.

Establishing evening rituals has been a game-changer for our family. Whether it's a shared dinner, reading a bedtime story, or simply sitting together and sharing highlights from our day, these rituals provide a sense of stability and togetherness that our children cherish. It's easy to get caught up in the hustle and bustle of daily life, but I've learned that prioritizing quality time with our family in the evening is essential. Even if it's just for a short period, those moments of focused attention can make a world of difference in building strong family bonds.

While routines are valuable, I've also learned the importance of flexibility and adaptability. Sometimes life throws unexpected curveballs, and it's okay to adjust our routines to accommodate the needs of the moment. The key is to remain open and responsive to the changing dynamics of family life.

Lastly, practicing mindful presence during our evening routines has been a powerful lesson. By being fully engaged in the moment, we can savor the simple joys of family life and create lasting memories. Mindfulness helps us appreciate the beauty in the ordinary.

Incorporating these lessons into our peaceful evening routines has not only strengthened our family bonds but has also allowed us to create a nurturing and harmonious home environment. It's a reminder that by setting aside screens and making intentional choices, we focus the space of the home for what truly matters: love, connection, and cherished moments with our family.

Reflection: Balancing Priorities

As you engaged in your mindful evening routine, you allowed yourself to step into a sacred space where work concerns were set aside, and the loving presence of your family took center stage. In the gentle embrace of this moment, you balanced the various priorities in your life and found solace in leaving work at work.

Here are some reflections on this balancing act:

1. **Leaving Work Behind:** The transition from work to home life can be challenging, but it's a crucial one. By consciously choosing to leave work at work and be fully present with your family, you demonstrate your commitment to your loved ones.

2. **Self-Care Matters:** Part of being present for your family is taking care of yourself. Your mindful evening routine allows you to recharge, ensuring that you have the energy and positivity to give to your family.

3. **Quality Over Quantity:** It's not about the quantity of time you spend with your family but the quality of the moments you share. These mindful moments are where connections are nurtured and bonds are strengthened.

4. **Gratitude:** Expressing gratitude for your family and the love that surrounds you is a powerful way to reinforce the importance of these relationships in your life.

5. **Balance and Harmony:** You're continually balancing your roles as a professional and a mother. Embracing mindful moments helps you find harmony and maintain a sense of equilibrium.

6. **Presence is a Gift:** Remember that your presence is a gift to your family. Being fully engaged with them, free from the distractions of work, shows your loved ones that they are your top priority.

7. **Boundaries:** Setting clear boundaries between work and personal life is an act of self-care. It allows you to protect your personal time and maintain a healthy work-life balance.

It takes significant discernment to navigate the delicate dance between your career and motherhood. By leaving work at work and embracing these mindful moments, you're fostering a nurturing and loving environment within your home—a gift that will resonate through generations to come.

Meditation: Embracing Mindful Moments

As your day winds down, find a quiet and cozy space in your home where you can sit comfortably. It could be a favorite chair, a spot by the window, or even your bed.

Take a few deep breaths, inhaling slowly through your nose and exhaling gently through your mouth. Allow the cares of the day to fall away with each exhale.

Close your eyes and bring your attention to the present moment.

Feel the weight of your body in the chair or on the bed, grounding yourself in the here and now.

Begin to notice the sounds around you—the soft hum of appliances, the distant laughter of your family members, or the calming rhythm of your breath.

Now, with your eyes still closed, picture your family members going about their evening routines.

Visualize their smiles, their actions, and the love that fills your home.

As you observe these moments, allow a sense of gratitude to wash over you.

You are blessed with a loving family and the opportunity to be a part of their lives.

Continue to focus on your breath as you repeat the following words in your mind: "I am present and mindful as I care for myself and my family."

Affirmation

"I am present and mindful as I care for myself and my family."

Repeat this affirmation, feeling it resonate within you, reminding you of the importance of being fully present in these cherished moments.

Imagine yourself wrapping each family member in a mental hug, sending them your love and appreciation.

By embracing mindful moments in your evening routine, you enhance your connection with your loved ones, fostering a deeper sense of love and appreciation within your family. Your presence is a gift that enriches not only your life but also the lives of those you hold dear

CHAPTER

04

Chapter 4: Balancing Work and Family

In the intricate dance of life, balancing the roles of a successful professional and a loving mother can be challenging. Mornings can be rough, and it often takes effort to keep work from intruding on our precious family time. But through mindfulness, we can find harmony in these dual roles.

Seeking Balance Amidst a Rough Morning

Imagine a day where everything that could have gone wrong did—alarm clock mishaps, spilled coffee, and missed deadlines. It felt like the whole day was destined for chaos. But in the midst of these challenges, let's explore how we can find balance and positivity to turn the day around.

Scene: It's early morning, and the mother's alarm clock fails to go off. She wakes up late, rushes to get herself ready, but in her haste, spills coffee on her work outfit. As she leaves for work, she's already feeling frazzled.

Mother (Thoughts): "This day is off to a terrible start. I'm late, and I've ruined my outfit. What else could possibly go wrong?"

Her Inner Voice: "Take a moment to pause. Yes, the morning didn't go as planned, but it doesn't define the entire day."

As the mother arrives at work, she faces a mountain of tasks and tight deadlines. It seems like the chaos from the morning is following her.

Mother (Thoughts): "I can't believe I'm behind on everything. This day is a disaster."

Her Inner Voice: "It's easy to dwell on the rough start, but remember, you have the power to change the course of your day."

During a lunch break, the mother takes a few minutes to practice deep breathing and refocus. She reminds herself of the balance she seeks between her roles.

Mother (Thoughts): "I may have had a rough morning, but I can still be a successful professional and a loving mother."

Her Inner Voice: "Exactly. Finding balance means acknowledging the imperfections of the morning and making the conscious choice to embrace positivity and balance in the present moment."

As the workday progresses, the mother finds small moments to connect with her colleagues, even amidst the chaos. She prioritizes her tasks, setting realistic goals, and leaves work at the office when it's time to head home.

Mother (Thoughts): "I can't control everything, but I can control how I react. I can be present for my family and make the most of the evening."

Her Inner Voice: "That's the spirit. By seeking balance in the midst of chaos, you're demonstrating resilience and strength."

As the mother arrives home, she tries to shrug off the challenges of the day, focusing on her family. She resets: despite the rough start, the mother chooses to focus on creating a positive and loving atmosphere at home.

Mother (Thoughts): "Today may have started off rocky, but it doesn't have to end that way. I can be present and make this evening special."

Her Inner Voice: "And in doing so, you bring balance and positivity to your family life, reminding yourself that it's not the challenges but how you respond to them that truly matters."

In this scenario, the mother's day began with chaos, but by seeking balance and positivity in each moment, she found the strength to turn things around. Life is filled with imperfections and rough starts, but our ability to find balance and positivity can transform even the most challenging days into opportunities for growth. Yet many of us struggle without that inner voice attuned to balance.

Meditation: Finding Harmony in Dual Roles

Begin by finding a quiet and comfortable place to sit or lie down.

Close your eyes and take a few deep breaths, allowing your body and mind to settle.

Imagine two sides of a scale, one representing your professional life and the other representing your role as a mother.

Visualize these scales in perfect balance, neither side tipping too far.

Now, think about a recent morning where things didn't go as planned.

Perhaps there was chaos, rushing, or frustration.

Acknowledge that such moments happen- they are part of life- and it's okay not to be perfect.

As you reflect on that challenging morning, picture it as a heavy weight on one side of the scale.

See it there, and allow it to represent the imperfections and challenges of life.

Slowly, begin to breathe deeply and evenly.

With each breath, imagine the weight of that challenging morning lifting, allowing the scale to find its balance once more.

As you focus on your breath, repeat the following affirmation: "I am a successful professional and a loving mother, in perfect balance."

Affirmation

"I am a successful professional and a loving mother, in perfect balance."

Visualize yourself going about your daily routines, smoothly transitioning from your professional life to your family life with grace and ease. See yourself as a loving mother who is also successful in her career.

Understand that it takes effort and intention to maintain this balance. Just as you release the weight of a challenging morning, remind yourself that you can also release the weight of work when you're with your family.

When you're ready, gently open your eyes, carrying this sense of balance and harmony with you into your daily life.

Balancing work and family is a constant journey filled with ups and downs. Life is imperfect, and rough mornings can happen. However, through mindfulness and the affirmation that you are a successful professional and a loving mother in perfect balance, you empower yourself to navigate these challenges.

Remember that perfection is not the goal; it's about finding harmony between your roles and making the effort to leave work behind when you're with your family. By doing so, you create a nurturing and loving environment for both your career and your loved ones.

CHAPTER 05

Chapter 5: Parenting with Patience

Parenting is a journey that requires patience, not just with our children, but also with ourselves and our partners. Let's explore how cultivating patience and understanding can lead to successful and fulfilling parenting.

Embracing Our Imperfect Patience

As we delve into the art of parenting with patience, it's essential to acknowledge the unique challenges faced by overstimulated mothers. Parenting is a demanding journey, and at times, our capacity for patience may feel limited. There are moments when we can practice patience and expand our capacity, but there are also times when we must make concessions before we lose our cool—because, in the end, we are only humans, doing our very best.

Motherhood, especially for those balancing the demands of work and family, often feels like a whirlwind of responsibilities, emotions, and constant stimulation. The world around us moves at a frantic pace, and it's easy to become overwhelmed.

In these moments, when we're stretched thin and feeling the weight of the world on our shoulders, our patience can wear thin. We may find ourselves on the brink of frustration or impatience, wondering if we're falling short of the ideal.

But let's remember this: practicing patience is not about being perfect; it's about making the conscious effort to embrace understanding and compassion, both for our children and ourselves.

There are days when we rise to the occasion, finding that reservoir of patience within us to guide our children through challenges with grace and kindness. These moments expand our capacity for patience, reminding us of our incredible strength.

However, there are also days when the chaos of life threatens to overwhelm us, when we feel our patience slipping away. In these moments, it's perfectly acceptable to make concessions, to acknowledge our limits, and to take a step back before we lose our cool.

Parenting is a journey of continuous learning and growth, one that doesn't come with a handbook of infallible answers. It's about navigating the unpredictable tides of life with love and resilience, recognizing that we, too, are human, subject to our emotions and limitations.

So, as we explore the practice of parenting with patience, let's remember that it's a journey marked by moments of success and moments of concession. It's a path where every effort to nurture our children with love and understanding is a triumph, no matter how imperfect it may seem.

In this chapter, we will delve into the art of finding balance, practicing patience, and embracing our imperfect nature as parents.

Meditation: Cultivating Patience and Understanding

Begin by finding a quiet and comfortable space to sit down. Close your eyes and take a few deep breaths, grounding yourself in the present moment.

Visualize yourself as a parent, navigating the beautiful but sometimes challenging journey of raising children.

Picture your children and your partner in this mental landscape.

As you breathe deeply, become aware of any impatience or frustration that may have arisen in your parenting journey.

Acknowledge that it's okay to feel these emotions but also recognize the power of patience in managing them.

Imagine a calm, nurturing light surrounding you, symbolizing patience. This light represents your ability to be patient with yourself, your children, and your partner.

Now, focus on yourself as a parent. Reflect on your own growth and learning process.

Visualize the times when you've made mistakes or felt overwhelmed, and allow yourself the grace to learn and grow from these experiences.

As you breathe, repeat the following words in your mind: "I am patient and understanding, nurturing my children with love."

Shift your focus to your children. Visualize them as individuals, each with their unique personalities and challenges.

See yourself as their guide, cultivating the patience and understanding to support them in their journey.

Consider your partner and their role in parenting. Recognize that they, too, have their moments of patience and impatience.

Visualize a bond of patience and understanding strengthening your partnership.

Affirmation

"I am patient and understanding, nurturing my children with love."

As you continue to breathe deeply, let go of any lingering impatience or frustration. Embrace a sense of calm and compassion for yourself, your children, and your partner.

When you're ready, slowly open your eyes, carrying this newfound sense of patience and understanding into your parenting journey.

Reflection

Parenting is a journey of growth, both for you and your children. It's a path that requires patience with yourself as you learn, patience with your children as they explore the world, and patience with your partner as you navigate this journey together.

Consider the following thoughts:

1. **Patience with Yourself:** Parenting is not about perfection but about growth. Be patient with yourself as you learn and adapt. Your love and intention matter most.
2. **Patience with Your Children:** Children are discovering the world, and they need your

patient guidance. Allow them to make mistakes and learn from them.

3. **Patience with Your Partner:** Parenting is a partnership. Open communication is essential to supporting each other with patience and understanding as you both navigate this shared journey.

4. **Cultivating Calm:** When impatience arises, pause, and take a deep breath. Remind yourself of your affirmation: "I am patient and understanding." This simple act can bring peace to challenging moments.

5. **Embracing Imperfection:** Know that you won't always get it right, and that's perfectly okay. Your patience and love are what truly matter in your children's lives.

By cultivating patience and understanding in your parenting journey, you create an environment of love and growth for yourself, your children, and your partner. This nurturing approach fosters resilience, empathy, and connection within your family, making your parenting journey all the more fulfilling and successful

CHAPTER
06

Chapter 6: Energizing Morning Ritual

In the journey of motherhood, it's easy to lose sight of our own well-being amidst the demands of family and work. Yet to nurture our children's vitality, we must first nourish our own. Let's explore the discipline required to develop lasting habits that support not only healthy motherhood but also our personal wellness.

As mothers, we're well-acquainted with the intricate dance of life's responsibilities. Each day, we step onto the stage, donning the many hats that motherhood demands. We run the show, a well-rehearsed drama that we do day in and day out. But it's during those brief morning hours that the stage is set, and the choices we make can profoundly impact the day ahead.

Mornings have a way of determining the course of our day—a delicate balance between maintaining our resolve and teetering on the brink of chaos. Let me take a moment to share from my personal experiences: the mornings when I chose to let go of the stressors that perennially plague me, as well as the ones where I wallowed in misery and too much caffeine. Finding balance internally is a journey, but it allows us to ride out those swirling, chaotic moments of parenthood.

The Rough Mornings

There are those mornings when sleep eludes us, our children are restless, or the alarm clock seems especially cruel. On such days, I've stood at the crossroads of my morning ritual. It's tempting to wallow in misery, to reach for that extra cup of caffeine, and to let the stress of the morning dictate my mood. I've juggled breakfast, daycare drop off routines, and work deadlines with a heavy heart, feeling like I'm already behind before the day begins. In these moments, I've struggled to find the resolve to prioritize my well-being amidst the chaos. And in the midst of that fleeting chaos, what even does it mean to care for myself, two little beings, a partner, and the rest of my life that needs me?

The Choice to Let Go

But then there are mornings when I've made a different choice—a choice to let go. On those days when sleep was fleeting and chaos seemed inevitable, I've embraced the imperfections of the morning. I've chosen to skip that extra cup of caffeine, to take a deep breath, and to remember that I am, after all, only human.

In doing so, I've set a different tone for the day, one filled with patience, self-compassion, and a sense of purpose. I've nurtured myself, allowing a few stolen moments of self-care, and have felt the profound impact this choice has on the day's unfolding.

Mornings have the remarkable power to make or break our resolve. They test our discipline, our patience, and our ability to balance the various balls we juggle as mothers. It's a dance that requires grace and determination, recognizing that each day is unique, and our mornings may be rough, smooth, or something in between.

Discipline in the Morning Ritual

In this chapter, we explore the discipline required to build lasting habits that support our wellness as individuals and as mothers. It's a journey that acknowledges the complexity of our lives and the delicacy of our balance. It's a journey that begins each morning when we choose to prioritize our well-being, no matter how rough the start may be.

Let us embark on this journey together, recognizing that we are all navigating the morning dance, striving to make the best choices for ourselves and our families. May we find the discipline to energize our mornings, setting a positive tone for the intricate balancing act that is motherhood.

Meditation: Setting Positive Intentions

Begin your morning ritual by finding a serene and uncluttered space where you can sit quietly. Close your eyes, take a deep breath, and allow the stresses of yesterday to fade away.

As you breathe deeply and evenly, envision a bright and radiant light filling your body.

This light symbolizes your energy and purpose for the day ahead.

Reflect on your identity as a mother and an individual.

Recognize that your energy and wellness are vital not only for your personal growth but also for your children's well-being.

Consider the habits you wish to cultivate in your morning routine. These could include meditation, exercise, journaling, or any activity that fills you with vitality.

As you contemplate these habits, set a positive intention for the day.

Visualize yourself as a beacon of energy and purpose, ready to embrace the challenges and joys that await.

Repeat the following affirmation: "I start each day with energy and purpose."

Affirmation

"I start each day with energy and purpose."

Imagine your day unfolding with intention and vitality. Visualize yourself engaging with your children, your work, and your own self-care with enthusiasm and vigor.

Take a few moments to acknowledge any resistance or obstacles that may arise in your journey to prioritize your well-being. Recognize that discipline is the key to building lasting habits that will energize your mornings.

When you're ready, gently open your eyes, carrying the sense of energy and purpose with you as you begin your day.

Reflection

Energizing your morning ritual is a disciplined choice that not only supports your healthy personhood but also enriches your capacity for healthy motherhood. Here are some thoughts that may help you develop this discipline:

1. **Prioritizing Self-Care:** By dedicating time to your own well-being in the morning, you are making a conscious choice to nurture yourself. This self-care is not selfish; it's essential for your overall health.

2. **Building Lasting Habits:** Discipline is the foundation for creating lasting habits. The more you practice energizing morning rituals, the more ingrained they become in your daily routine.
3. **Leading by Example:** As you prioritize your wellness, you set an example for your children. They learn the importance of self-care and healthy habits by observing your choices.
4. **Sustaining Energy:** When you start your day with purpose and vitality, you are better equipped to face the challenges and joys of motherhood. Your energy ripples through your interactions with your family.
5. **Balance and Boundaries:** Discipline involves setting boundaries to protect your morning routine. It's a way of respecting your own needs and priorities.
6. **Embracing Imperfection:** There will be days when discipline wavers, and that's perfectly normal. Embrace these moments as opportunities for growth, not as failures.

Your intention to start each day with purpose sets a positive tone for your journey as both an individual and a mother, enriching both your own life and the lives of your loved ones.

CHAPTER 07

Chapter 7: Mindful Breathing for Moms

In the whirlwind of motherhood, it's easy to lose touch with our inner selves. Yet, amidst the chaos, we can find solace and grounding through the simple act of mindful breathing. This chapter explores the importance of staying connected to our inner selves through breath and introduces grounding and restorative breathing techniques that are accessible even to the busiest of mothers.

Staying Connected to My Breath

In the midst of my busy days as a mother, work, and life's constant demands, I've come to realize the incredible impact of staying connected to my breath. It's a practice that not only helps me re-center after meetings but also serves as a lifeline to my inner self, guiding me through life's storms. Too often do I realize that I have been tense for hours, perhaps all day, without letting breath flow through my body.

Re-centering After Meetings

Meetings often leave me with a swirl of thoughts, emotions, and a sense of being pulled in different directions. It's in those moments when I find solace in reconnecting with my breath. I step away, find a quiet corner, and take a few deep breaths. As I inhale and exhale intentionally, I can feel the tension from the meeting dissipate. My mind clears, and I regain perspective.

Breathing becomes my anchor, a reminder that no matter how chaotic or challenging a meeting may be, I have the power to return to a place of calm and focus. It's a simple yet profoundly effective way to transition from one task to the next, ready to face whatever comes my way with a sense of grace.

The Effects of Losing Connection

On the flip side, there have been moments when I've unintentionally disconnected from my breath, holding it as if bracing for impact during times of stress. This is when I've felt tension building in my body, like a coiled spring ready to snap. It's as if I've temporarily lost touch with the rhythm of life.

In those moments, my emotional capacity feels constrained. I become reactive rather than responsive. I'm more prone to impatience and frustration, unable to access the reservoir of patience and understanding within me. It's as if I'm running on empty, and my ability to nurture my children and myself is compromised. In the end, losing connection to myself causes me to lose ability to support my little beings.

The Lifeline of Breath

Recognizing the power of breath has been a game-changer. It's a lifeline to my inner self, a reminder that I have the capacity to choose how I respond to life's challenges. Whether it's taking a few deep breaths during a hectic day or deliberately breathing through a stressful moment, staying connected to my breath grounds me.

Breathing is a testament to my resilience, a practice that has helped me weather the storms of motherhood and daily life. It's a gentle yet potent reminder that, no matter how chaotic life may become, I can find calm within by simply reconnecting with my breath.

So, I make every attempt to continue to breathe intentionally throughout my day. I take those precious moments to re-center, to nurture my emotional capacity, and to remind myself that, as a mother, I possess an inner wellspring of strength and serenity, accessible with every mindful breath I take. If I give myself the space to continue breathing, to stay connected to my whole self-body and mind, I have more connection and ability to respond to every-day stressors vs. reacting from a place of disconnection.

Meditation: Deep Breathing for Relaxation

Begin by finding a comfortable and quiet space where you can sit or lie down. Close your eyes and take a moment to settle into the present moment.

Bring your attention to your breath.

Take a slow, deep breath in through your nose, allowing your abdomen to rise as you fill your lungs.

Exhale slowly and completely through your mouth, feeling any tension or stress leaving your body.

Continue this deep breathing pattern, inhaling for a count of four and exhaling for a count of six.

With each breath, imagine a sense of calm and relaxation washing over you.

As you continue to breathe deeply, visualize yourself in a peaceful and serene place, whether it's a tranquil beach, a serene forest, or a cozy corner of your home.

Repeat the following affirmation in your mind: "I breathe deeply and find calm within."

Affirmation

"I breathe deeply and find calm within."

Feel the calming energy of this affirmation enveloping you as you regulate your breathing.

If your mind begins to wander, gently bring your focus back to your breath and the affirmation, allowing any distractions to melt away.

After several minutes of deep breathing and affirmation, slowly open your eyes, feeling refreshed and centered.

Exploring Grounding and Restorative Breathing Techniques

In the hustle and bustle of daily life, finding moments for mindful breathing is essential. Here are a few techniques to explore that will allow u to stay connected to your breathing in the midst of the busiest of schedules:

1. **Grounding Breath:** When you feel overwhelmed or anxious, try grounding breath. Inhale deeply through your nose for a count of four, hold your breath for a count of four, and then exhale through your mouth for a count of six. This technique helps bring you back to the present moment.

2. **Morning Reset:** Start your day with a few minutes of deep, intentional breathing. Inhale deeply as you wake up, visualizing positive energy filling your body, and exhale any lingering sleepiness.

3. Evening Calm: Before bed, practice deep breathing and affirmation to release the day's stresses and prepare your mind and body for restful sleep.

4. **Micro-Breathing:** Incorporate short moments of deep breathing throughout your day, even during tasks like cooking or working. Take a few deep breaths to reset and re-center yourself.

5. **Mindful Breaks:** Whenever possible, steal moments for a quick deep-breathing session, whether it's while waiting for your child, during a coffee break, or before an important meeting.

Incorporating mindful breathing into your daily routine can help you stay connected to your inner self, find moments of calm amidst the chaos, and nurture your overall well-being. By prioritizing your breath, you ground and center yourself to face the challenges and joys of each day with clarity and serenity.

CHAPTER 08

Chapter 8: Letting Go of Mom Guilt

Motherhood is a complex journey, filled with joy, love, and profound moments. Yet, it's also a landscape riddled with psychological, emotional, societal, and internal pressures, often leading to the all-too-familiar feeling of maternal guilt. In this chapter, we'll delve into the impossible cocktail of expectations that contribute to this guilt and offer a meditation to help you release it, along with an affirmation to embrace self-compassion.

Embrace Imperfection and Release Expectations

The journey of motherhood is a winding path, filled with both breathtaking vistas and challenging terrain. Amidst this journey, one truth has become crystal clear to me: the expectations we carry, whether internal or external, are an impossible burden, even the ones we set for ourselves.

I want to share another personal story on the ever-present weight of expectations, the value of normalizing self-disappointment, and the imperative need to desensitize ourselves to external guilt factors. None of us are immune to the social, generational, cultural, and familial burdens of expectation. This might be one of the unifying factors across race and class for mothers- the challenge of impossible expectations.

Normalizing the Impossible Burden of Expectations & Self Disappointment

It's natural to have expectations, and as mothers, we often set the bar impossibly high. The standards we hold for ourselves can become a relentless quest for perfection, a quest that ultimately leaves us feeling inadequate and guilty. The expectations imposed upon us from external sources, be it society, family, or friends, only add to this already towering burden.

One of the most profound lessons motherhood has taught me is the art of normalizing self-disappointment. Yes, you read that right—normalizing it. It's the understanding that perfection is an illusion, and there will be moments of falling short, of not living up to my own expectations. Instead of beating myself up over these moments, I've learned to acknowledge them as part of the human experience.

Developing a Thick Skin to External Guilt

In our journey as mothers, we often find ourselves in the crossfire of external guilt factors—societal judgments, well-meaning advice, and the scrutiny of others. Desensitizing ourselves to these external voices is essential. It means recognizing that we cannot control what others think or say, but we can control how much power we give to their opinions.

Perfection is an unattainable ideal, a mirage that leads us away from the genuine experience of motherhood. The truth is, we are beautifully imperfect beings doing our best. Normalizing self-disappointment and desensitizing to external guilt factors frees us from the relentless pursuit of perfection and allows us to embrace the beauty of our imperfections.

In the chapters that follow, we will explore the power of self-compassion and self-acceptance. We'll delve into techniques that help us release guilt, both self-imposed and external, and create a space for love and understanding. Remember, self-compassion is not just an aspiration but a practice—an act of kindness that we extend to ourselves in moments of self-disappointment.

So, as you journey through this chapter, I invite you to reflect on the expectations you carry, the self-disappointment you may have felt, and the external guilt factors that have touched your life. Know that you are not alone in this experience. As mothers, we almost have to accept that that our self-expectations are skewed by factors beyond our control. Perhaps we should expect to disappoint ourselves since we are measuring by a skewed scale? By embracing imperfection and normalizing self-disappointment, we take the first steps toward releasing the heavy burden of guilt and finding freedom in self-compassion.

The Impossible Cocktail of Expectations

Motherhood carries a weighty burden of expectations—psychological, emotional, societal, and internal—all mixed into an impossible cocktail that mothers are served daily. The psychological pressure to be perfect, the emotional rollercoaster of trying to balance it all, societal judgments, and our internalized expectations create a perfect storm for maternal guilt.

1. **Psychological Pressure:** Society often perpetuates an idealized image of motherhood, where mothers are expected to be selfless, nurturing, and endlessly patient. We're told that any deviation from this ideal is a failure, breeding guilt.
2. **Emotional Balancing Act:** Juggling work, family, and personal life can be emotionally taxing. We strive to give our best in every sphere, but the fear of falling short can stir up guilt when we can't be everywhere at once.
3. **Societal Judgments:** Mothers often face judgments from society and even other mothers. Choices regarding breastfeeding,

education, discipline, and career are scrutinized, and these judgments fuel maternal guilt.

4. **Internalized Expectations:** Perhaps the most insidious source of guilt is the expectations we place on ourselves. We're our own harshest critics, constantly questioning if we're doing enough or doing it right.

Meditation: Releasing Guilt and Embracing Self-Compassion

Find a quiet and comfortable space to sit or lie down. Close your eyes, and take a few deep breaths, allowing your body to relax.

Visualize the weight of mom guilt as a heavy burden you've been carrying.

See it clearly in your mind's eye, feel how much this guilt has cost you of your self-worth.

Imagine this burden slowly lifting from your shoulders, becoming lighter with each breath you take.

As you continue to breathe deeply, picture a warm and soothing light surrounding you.

This light represents self-compassion and understanding; understanding that the expectations you have been measuring against are in fact impossible.

Let the light enlighten your expectations of yourself, separating them from those that are unrealistic of any mother.

You are free of that weight. Any guilt that creeps into your mind after this time—it is the ghost of false beliefs haunting you.

Repeat the following affirmation: "I am a loving mother, free from guilt and full of self-compassion."

Affirmation

"I am a loving mother, free from guilt and full of self-compassion."

Allow the self-compassion to envelop you, like a loving embrace, as you release the burden of guilt.

Visualize yourself as a mother who loves, nurtures, and makes choices based on love, not fear or guilt. See yourself as enough, just as you are.

If feelings of guilt arise during this meditation, acknowledge them with kindness and then gently release them, returning to the affirmation of self-compassion.

Reflection

Maternal guilt is a heavy burden, one that many of us carry without realizing its destructive power. In this chapter, we've explored the myriad expectations placed upon mothers from various sources. We've acknowledged the guilt that stems from trying to meet these expectations and the pressure we place on ourselves. Consider the following thoughts:

1. **You Are Enough:** It's essential to recognize that you are enough just as you are. You love your children, and you're doing your best.
2. **Letting Go:** Releasing guilt doesn't mean giving up on growth or self-improvement. It means letting go of the unreasonable expectations that weigh you down.
3. **Self-Compassion:** Embrace self-compassion as a guiding light on your journey of motherhood. Be as kind to yourself as you are to your children.
4. **Community:** Seek a supportive community of mothers who understand the challenges you face. Sharing experiences and support can alleviate guilt.

5. **Choices Made with Love:** Recognize that your choices are made with love, even if they don't align with societal norms or someone else's expectations.

As you journey through motherhood, remember that letting go of mom guilt is an act of self-compassion. By releasing this burden, you create space for joy, self-love, and a more fulfilling experience as a mother.

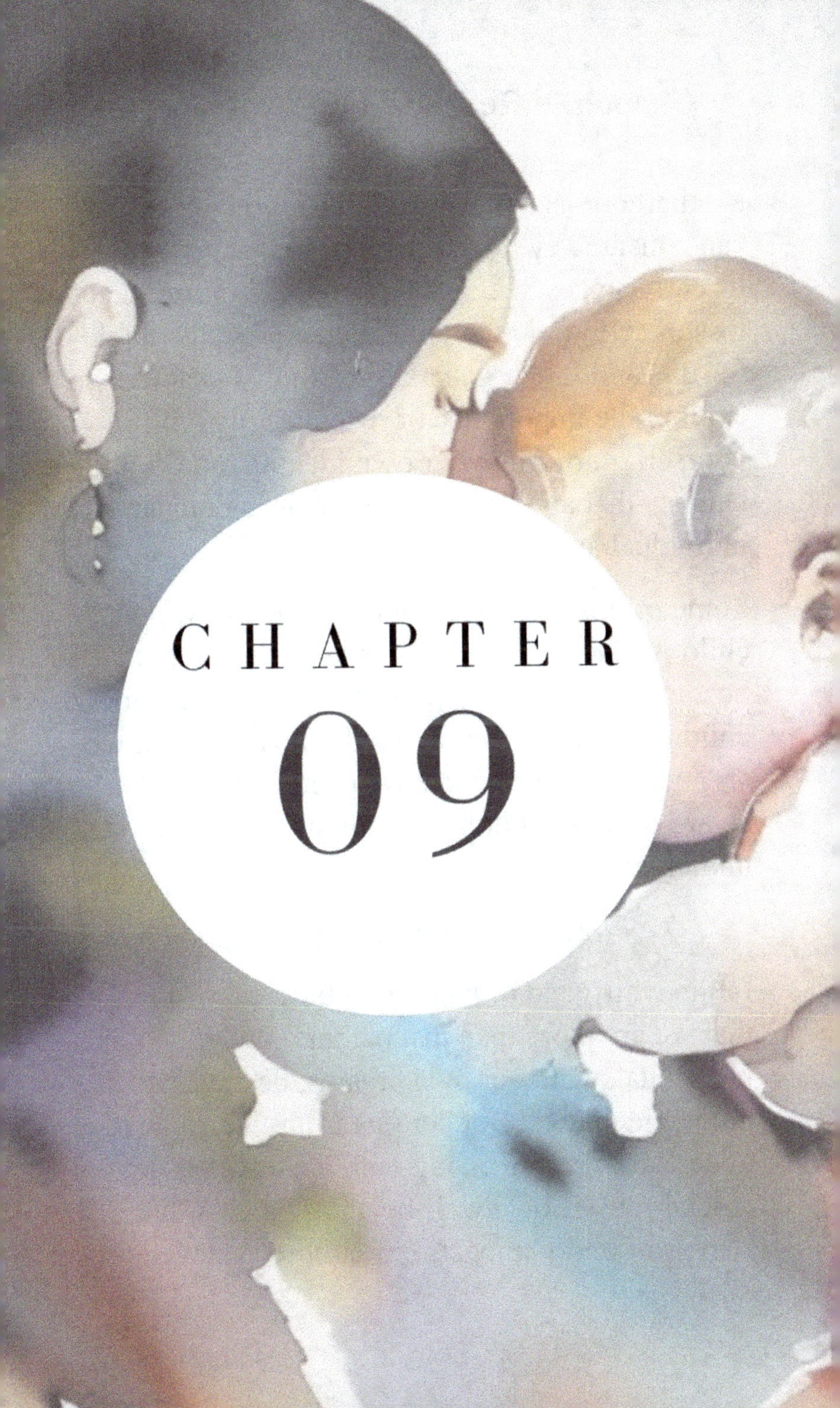
CHAPTER
09

Chapter 9: Reconnecting with Yourself

Motherhood is a transformative journey, one that can consume every fiber of our being, especially in its early stages. Yet, it's crucial to recognize that the loss of self in motherhood need not be inevitable for this and future generations. In this chapter, we explore the importance of reconnecting with yourself, nurturing your own identity, and finding a balance that allows you to flourish as both an individual and a parent.

Some of this reconnection is with the raw inner child wounds for our own growing up years that become abundantly apparent when raising our own children. In early motherhood, the time when we are most acutely needed, we become painfully aware of those childhood wounds due to our own unmet needs.

The Power of Reconnecting with Ourselves

In the whirlwind of parenthood, it's easy to forget that we are more than just parents. We are individuals with our own dreams, desires, and unique identities. But here's a truth I've come to understand: reconnecting with ourselves is not only crucial for our own well-being as parents, but it also profoundly impacts our children's development and the strength of the partnership we forge with our co-parent or life partner.

In this chapter, we'll delve into the transformative journey of rediscovering our own identities and how this journey ripples through every aspect of our lives.

Parental Well-Being & Child Development

As parents, we often put our children's needs before our own, and while this is a noble act, it can sometimes lead to neglecting our own identities. Reconnecting with ourselves isn't selfish; it's a vital step toward becoming happier, more fulfilled parents.

When we nurture our own identities alongside our roles as parents, we set a powerful example for our children. We show them the importance of self-discovery, independence, and pursuing their passions. In doing so, we support their healthy development.

Reconnecting with ourselves also strengthens the partnership we share with our co-parent or life partner. By nurturing our own needs and desires, we become more balanced individuals and, in turn, contribute to a more harmonious

and supportive partnership. So, as you embark on this chapter, keep in mind that reconnecting with yourself isn't just about you—it's a gift you give to your children and a building block for a stronger, more fulfilling partnership. It's a journey toward becoming the best version of yourself, both as an individual and as a parent.

All-Consuming Season of Early Motherhood

Early motherhood is an intense season of life. The demands of caring for a newborn, sleepless nights, and the constant attention required can easily lead to the feeling of being engulfed by motherhood. It's a season of profound love and care, but it can also be a time when our own identity gets eclipsed.

Losing oneself entirely in motherhood can have unintended consequences. It may lead to an unhealthy parenting style, where we seek fulfillment primarily through our children. In doing so, we might inadvertently burden our children with our unmet needs, hindering their ability to develop a sense of self and independence.

Reconnecting with yourself doesn't mean neglecting your responsibilities as a mother. Instead, it's about recognizing that your identity and needs matter alongside your role as a parent. It's about nurturing your own desires, dreams, and interests alongside those of your children.

Meditation: Rediscovering Your Inner Self

Find a comfortable and quiet space where you can sit or lie down. Close your eyes gently, and take a few deep, cleansing breaths. Allow yourself to be fully present in this moment.

As a mother, especially during the all-consuming season of early motherhood, it's easy to lose sight of your own needs and desires. Today, we embark on a journey to rediscover your inner self, to nurture the woman within the mother.

Let's embrace stillness for a moment: Imagine yourself in a serene, tranquil garden.

This garden represents your inner world—a place of beauty and introspection.

As you walk through this garden, notice the gentle rustle of leaves and the calming sounds of nature.

Take a moment to embrace the stillness within you.

Inhale deeply, and as you exhale, release any tension or distractions.

This is your sacred space to explore your inner self, including reflection on interests and passions you engaged in prior to becoming a mother.

In this garden, you encounter a quiet, secluded area where you can sit and reflect.

Think back to the passions and interests that defined you before motherhood.

What activities or hobbies brought you joy and fulfillment?

As you reminisce, allow the memories of those passions to envelop you like a warm embrace. Remember the sense of purpose and happiness these interests brought into your life.

Now, shift your focus to the present moment.

What desires and dreams reside within you, waiting to be awakened or rekindled?

Visualize these desires as radiant stars within your inner sky, each one representing a unique aspiration.

Choose one desire that calls to you the most. See it shine brightly within your inner garden.

This desire represents your personal journey of rediscovery.

In the midst of your nurturing journey, let's also remember the importance of self-care.

Visualize a gentle stream flowing through your inner garden.

This stream symbolizes self-care—a source of nourishment and rejuvenation.

Dip your hands into the crystal-clear waters and feel the soothing energy of self-care revitalizing you.

It's a reminder that nurturing yourself is essential to nurturing others.

Affirm yourself: "I embrace the journey of rediscovering my inner self.

My passions and desires are like guiding stars, lighting my path.

Through self-care and introspection, I nurture both the mother and the woman within me."

Take a moment to savor the serenity of this inner garden and the intentions you've set.

When you're ready, gently open your eyes, carrying with you the commitment to honor your passions, desires, and the importance of self-care as you continue your journey of rediscovery.

Affirmation

"I reconnect with myself, nurturing my own needs and desires."

Embrace the idea that by nurturing your own identity, you become a more fulfilled and well-rounded individual, capable of providing a healthier, balanced, and more nurturing environment for your children.

Take a moment to acknowledge any resistance or guilt that may arise. Understand that nurturing your identity is not selfish; it's a way to become a more present and nurturing parent.

When you're ready, open your eyes, carrying with you the sense of reconnecting with yourself.

Reflection

Reconnecting with yourself is not a selfish endeavor; it's a necessary one:

1. **Balancing Act:** By nurturing your own needs and desires, you create a healthy balance between your role as a mother and your identity as an individual.
2. **Modeling Independence:** Showing your children that you prioritize your own well-being and interests sets a valuable example of independence.
3. **Healthy Parenting:** Reconnecting with yourself leads to healthier parenting. When you are fulfilled and grounded, you are better equipped to nurture your children's needs without overburdening them with your own.
4. **Time for Self:** Finding time for yourself is not about taking time away from your children but about rejuvenating yourself so you can be a more present and patient parent.
5. **Unleash Potential:** Reconnecting with yourself may unlock hidden talents, passions,

and dreams, which can bring new purpose and joy to your life.

Reconnecting with yourself is a gift you give not only to yourself but also to your children. It's an acknowledgment that you are more than just a parent—you are a unique individual with your own desires and dreams. By nurturing your own identity, you create a harmonious space where your children can explore their own needs and desires with the support and guidance of a wholehearted and fulfilled parent.

CHAPTER 10

Chapter 10: Mindful Bedtime Routines

Bedtime is a cherished part of parenting. It's a time when we lovingly guide our children through the transitions from the wakeful world to the peaceful realm of dreams. We put careful thought and effort into our children's bedtime routines, knowing that these rituals provide comfort and structure. Yet, it's equally crucial to recognize that as parents, we need to re-parent ourselves into a psychologically safe and regulated place to create a similarly safe and regulated space for our children.

My Struggles with Sleep Regulation

As I sit down to write about the importance of a mindful bedtime routine, I can't help but reflect on my own journey with sleep. It's been a journey marked by hyper vigilance, insomnia, and the echoes of my parents' unmet needs that still reverberate through the decades.

In my early years, sleep wasn't just a nightly ritual; it was a battleground. Hyper vigilance—a heightened state of alertness that's often a response to trauma—cast a shadow over my nights. The simplest creak of a floorboard or rustle of leaves outside my window would send my heart racing. I'd lie awake, my mind racing in tandem with my heartbeat, convinced that danger lurked just beyond the darkness.

Insomnia became a close companion during those years. The more I craved sleep, the more elusive it became. Countless nights were spent tossing and turning, trapped in a relentless cycle of anxiety, restlessness, and sleeplessness.

Yet, the roots of my sleep struggles stretched even further back, entwined with my parents' unmet needs from their own childhoods. As a child, I was keenly aware of their insecurities, their unspoken fears, and their unmet desires. I internalized their emotions, as children often do, believing it was my role to fill the voids in their lives.

As I grew older, the weight of these unmet needs lingered, morphing into a constant companion that accompanied me into adulthood. Despite my best efforts to free myself from this psychological baggage, I found that the specters of my past still haunted my sleep.

The path to reclaiming a healthy relationship with sleep has been anything but linear. It has involved years of self-reflection, therapy, and a commitment to re-parent myself into a place of psychological safety and regulation. While it's a journey that continues to this day, I've learned some invaluable lessons.

First and foremost, I've come to understand that healing is a gradual process, and that self-compassion is an essential part of that journey. I've learned to treat myself with the same kindness and understanding that I would offer to a dear friend.

I've also discovered the power of mindfulness and relaxation techniques, which have helped calm my overactive mind and guide me into a state of relaxation before bedtime. And yes, I've embraced the importance of a mindful bedtime routine, not only for my children but for myself.

As I write these words, I'm acutely aware of the progress I've made and the steps I continue to take toward a more peaceful night's sleep. I share this personal aside not as a testament to my struggles, but as a reminder that the journey to healthy sleep and regulation can be complex and deeply rooted in our past.

In this chapter, we explore the beauty of a mindful bedtime routine—one that extends beyond our children to nurture our own well-being. It's a reminder that by prioritizing our own sleep hygiene, we create a safe and regulated space within us, allowing us to provide the same for our children.

Remember, it's never too late to embark on a journey toward healthier sleep patterns and inner peace. It's a journey I'm grateful to be on, and one that offers hope to all who seek a restful night's sleep, no matter what challenges they may face

Re-Parenting Ourselves & Psychological Safety

Bedtime can be a battleground in parenthood. From sleepless nights with newborns to the burgeoning independence of toddlers, the journey to a restful night's sleep can be filled with challenges. Yet, we persevere, creating routines that help our children find comfort, security, and the serenity they need to drift into slumber.

In the process of nurturing our children's bedtime routines, we often come face to face with our own inner child—the one who may have struggled with fear of the dark or the vulnerability of sleep. This realization opens a door to the importance of re-parenting ourselves.

Re-parenting ourselves isn't just about addressing past fears; it's also about creating a psychologically safe and regulated space within us. By tending to our own sleep hygiene and well-being, we not only care for ourselves but also become better-equipped parents who can provide the same safety and regulation for our children. Whether it's a white noise machine, blackout shades, or a sleep podcast with a bedtime story to soothe yourself to sleep, those are legitimate needs.

Meditation: Preparing for Restful Sleep

Find a comfortable and quiet space in your bedroom. Dim the lights and create a peaceful atmosphere. Lie down on your back with your arms by your sides and your legs slightly apart. Close your eyes and take a deep breath in, exhaling slowly. Allow yourself to fully relax.

Begin by focusing on your breath. Inhale deeply through your nose, counting to three. Exhale slowly through your mouth, counting to four. Feel the tension leaving your body with each breath.

Visualize a radiant sunset on the horizon, symbolizing the end of your day's activities. As you watch the sun slowly set, imagine any worries or stressors being absorbed by the setting sun's warm glow.

Imagine your bedroom as a sanctuary of serenity, protected by a shimmering light. Feel the comfort of your bed and pillow. This is your safe haven.

Think of three things you're grateful for from today. Repeat this affirmation: "I release the day's worries, grateful for its blessings. I embrace restful sleep with an open heart."

Imagine yourself floating on a cloud of tranquility, becoming more relaxed with each breath.

Let go of tension in your muscles and drift deeper into relaxation.

Trust that you are fully prepared for restorative sleep.

Take one last deep breath and exhale fully. Surrender to the peaceful embrace of sleep. Goodnight, and sleep well.

Affirmation

"I am at peace, ready to embrace a restful night's sleep."

As you continue to breathe deeply and repeat the affirmation, let go of any worries or anxieties. Release any tension in your body.

Acknowledge the importance of prioritizing your own sleep hygiene, knowing that by doing so, you create a safe and regulated space within yourself and in your home.

When you're ready, slowly open your eyes, feeling rejuvenated and ready for a peaceful night's sleep.

Reflection

Prioritizing your own sleep hygiene is an act of self-care that benefits both you and your children. Here are some thoughts to consider:

1. **Creating a Sleep Sanctuary:** Design your bedroom as a serene sanctuary, a place of comfort and tranquility where you can recharge.
2. **Consistent Bedtime Routine:** Just as you create a bedtime routine for your children, establish one for yourself. Consistency helps signal to your body that it's time to wind down.
3. **Unplug:** Turn off electronic devices at least an hour before bedtime to allow your mind to relax.
4. **Mindful Preparation:** Prepare your mind and body for sleep by engaging in calming activities such as reading, gentle stretching, or meditation.
5. **Self-Compassion:** If you have trouble falling asleep, practice self-compassion. Be patient with yourself, knowing that sleep is a natural process that sometimes requires time and care.

Remember, as you tend to your own sleep hygiene, you create a loving and regulated space for your children to find comfort and security. It's a harmonious cycle where your well-being enriches theirs, and their serenity nourishes your own. While our children may need us at night, interrupting our rest, these phases are short-lived.

CHAPTER
11

Chapter 11: Embracing Imperfection

In the grand tapestry of parenthood, one thread stands out prominently: imperfection. While we strive to be the best parents we can be, it's essential to recognize that making mistakes is part of the journey. What truly matters is how we acknowledge, learn from, and repair relationships after those inevitable missteps. In this chapter, we explore the beauty of embracing imperfection and offer a meditation and affirmation to guide us on this path.

My Journey with Overstimulation and Reactivity

As I write about the importance of embracing imperfection in parenting, I can't help but think about a chapter of my own journey—one that's marked by moments of overstimulation and reactions that I'm not proud of. These moments have, at times, left a significant impact on my relationship with my children.

There have been moments when I've yelled at my children out of my own overstimulation. Times when the noise and chaos of the world, both internal and external, seemed to converge into a deafening cacophony. Those were the moments when I felt like I was losing control, that my patience was hanging by a thread, and that I had to release the pent-up tension somehow.

And so, I yelled. My words, laced with frustration and impatience, landed like a heavy blow. I saw the hurt in my children's eyes, and it cut deep. I felt an immediate pang of regret, followed by guilt that clung to me like a shadow. These reactions, born out of my own struggles with overstimulation, left a mark on our relationship—a mark I knew I had to address.

My journey toward embracing imperfection began with an acknowledgment of these moments. I realized that I couldn't erase them or pretend they didn't happen. Instead, I had to confront them with honesty and humility.

I started by owning my mistakes. I sat down with my children and apologized. I looked them in the eyes and told them that I was sorry for raising my voice, for letting my frustration spill over onto them. It was a difficult but necessary step.

But apologies, I've learned, are only a starting point. True change required me to dig deeper, to explore the roots of my overstimulation and reactivity. I sought support from therapists and counselors who helped me understand the triggers that pushed me over the edge.

Slowly, I began to cultivate a practice of self-regulation. I learned techniques to calm my mind and body in moments of overstimulation. I discovered the power of mindfulness, of taking a pause before reacting. It wasn't easy, and I'm still on this journey, but I've made progress.

What I've come to understand is that embracing imperfection isn't about avoiding mistakes altogether. It's about how we respond to those mistakes. It's about taking responsibility for our reactions and using them as opportunities for growth.

I'm learning to create a space for my children—one where I will own my mistakes and apologize when needed. But more than that, I've worked to shift my behavior. I've strived to create an environment where my children feel safe, loved, and heard. Though my children are still young, I am seeing the impact of these changes. Our relationship has deepened, and my children have learned a valuable lesson—not just in forgiveness but in resilience and empathy. They've learned that even parents make mistakes, but it's how we respond to those mistakes that defines us.

So I share with you not from a place of perfection but from a place of experience. I've learned that imperfection is not a stain on our parenting journey as parents; it's the canvas on which we paint the masterpiece of a relationship with our children. It's a canvas that allows for growth, compassion, and the ever-evolving dance of parenthood.

The Paradox of Parenting

Parenthood is an intricate dance of love, patience, and resilience. Despite our best intentions, we are not infallible. We make mistakes. We lose our temper. We stumble and falter. But in this dance, it's not the perfection of our steps that matters most; it's our willingness to acknowledge our missteps and continue the dance with grace and humility.

Acknowledging our imperfections is the first step in this dance. It means recognizing when we've erred, whether it's a harsh word spoken in frustration or a momentary lapse in patience. Owning our slip-ups opens the door to repair, a process that can strengthen the bonds between parent and child.

Mistakes, when viewed as opportunities for growth, become valuable lessons. They teach us patience, humility, and the importance of forgiveness—both toward ourselves and our children. Each mistake is a chance to refine our parenting skills and deepen our understanding of ourselves and our children.

Meditation: Embracing the Beauty of Imperfection

Find a quiet and comfortable space where you can sit or lie down. Close your eyes and take a deep breath in, exhaling slowly. Allow yourself to settle into a state of relaxation.

Begin by focusing on your breath. Inhale deeply through your nose, counting to three. Exhale slowly through your mouth, counting to four. Feel the tension leaving your body with each breath.

Visualize a beautiful garden, filled with a variety of flowers. Notice how each flower is unique, with its own imperfections and quirks. Embrace the imperfections of these flowers as part of their beauty.

Let's reflect on your as a mother. Recall moments when you felt imperfect or made mistakes. See these moments as stepping stones in your growth and learning. Understand that imperfection is a part of the beautiful mosaic of your life.

Place your hand on your heart and repeat the following affirmation: "I am a good mother, despite my imperfections.

I love and accept myself as I am." Feel the warmth of self-compassion filling your heart.

Imagine your child as they are, with all their growing edges and uniqueness.

See their beauty in every quirk and flaw. Know that your acceptance and love nurture their self-worth.

Take a deep breath in and exhale slowly. Carry the awareness of imperfection's beauty with you as you go about your day.

Embrace the imperfect moments as opportunities for growth and connection.

You are a beautiful mother, imperfectly perfect in every way.

Affirmation

"I am a good mother, despite my imperfections."

Feel the weight of self-compassion and acceptance wash over you. You are a loving parent, even in moments of imperfection.

Think about a specific parenting mistake you've made recently. Instead of dwelling on guilt, focus on the lessons you can learn and how you can repair any emotional wounds it may have caused.

As you continue to breathe mindfully, extend the same compassion you offer to yourself to your child. Imagine a loving conversation where you acknowledge the mistake and express your love and commitment to repair any harm.

When you're ready, gently open your eyes, carrying the affirmation and the beauty of your imperfections with you.

Reflection

Embracing imperfection is a profound act of self-compassion and love. Here are some thoughts to consider:

1. **Repair and Reconnect:** Repairing relationships after mistakes can deepen the trust and bond between you and your child. Apologize sincerely and demonstrate your commitment to positive change.
2. **Lessons from Mistakes:** Reflect on the specific parenting mistakes you've made. What have you learned from them? How can you apply these lessons to become a more understanding and patient parent?
3. **Forgiving Yourself:** Self-forgiveness is a crucial aspect of embracing imperfection. Remember that you are not defined by your mistakes; you are defined by your efforts to grow and learn from them.

4. **Humility and Growth:** Acknowledging your imperfections with humility opens the door to growth and self-improvement. It's a powerful demonstration of the love you have for your child and for yourself.

5. **The Beauty of Uniqueness**: Just as imperfections make every object unique and beautiful, your imperfections make you a unique and loving parent. Embrace your uniqueness and cherish it as part of your parenting journey.

In the tapestry of parenthood, imperfections are not flaws; they are the intricate patterns that give depth and character to the fabric of your relationship with your child. Embracing these imperfections with love, humility, and the commitment to learn and repair is what truly defines the beauty of your journey as a parent.

CHAPTER

12

Chapter 12: Boosting Self-Confidence

In the cacophony of societal pressures, the relentless march of parental stress, and the myriad challenges that parenthood presents, it's all too easy to find ourselves in a place where our maternal self-confidence has taken a beating. The weight of these pressures can lead to anxiety and depression, often tempting us to check out of the parenting game—whether through excessive phone use, a bit too much wine, or overindulgence in caffeine. In this chapter, we explore the art of boosting self-confidence, offering a meditation and affirmation to help you rebuild your belief in yourself as a mother.

Becoming Your Own Best Cheerleader

In the world of motherhood, it's easy to find ourselves relying on the evaluations and judgments of others. We seek validation from friends, partners, and even society at large, hoping to hear that we're doing a good job. And while external support is undoubtedly valuable, there's a truth we must embrace: true self-confidence can only come from our determination to relate to ourselves.

We live in a world that often measures our worth by external standards. It tells us how we should look, what we should achieve, and even how we should mother. We internalize these messages, making it all too easy to seek approval from others, to let their evaluations dictate our sense of self-worth.

But let me share a powerful insight I've gained on this journey: being your own best cheerleader is not a luxury; it's a necessity. While supportive friends and partners are wonderful allies on this path, they cannot replace the unwavering support that comes from within.

Self-confidence, that deep and unshakable belief in your abilities as a mother, arises from your own determination to relate to yourself with kindness, understanding, and compassion. It means looking inside, examining your thoughts and feelings, and forging a connection with the remarkable woman and mother that you are.

It's not always easy. In fact, at times, it can be incredibly challenging. It's tempting to avoid turning that introspective gaze inward. It's easier to distract ourselves with external validation, whether it's a pat on the back from a friend or the likes on a social media post.

But I urge you to resist that temptation, because the most important relationship you'll ever have is the one you have with yourself. It's the relationship that forms the foundation of all others, including your relationship with your children.

In a world that often celebrates perfection and glosses over imperfections, it's crucial that we don't lose our connection to ourselves. Embrace the moments of introspection, the times when you look in the mirror, not to scrutinize, but to appreciate the strength and beauty within.

Celebrate your achievements, no matter how small they may seem. Forgive your mistakes, for they are the stepping stones of growth. And above all, be your own biggest advocate, your most fervent supporter, and your loudest cheerleader.

Remember, self-confidence is not about becoming someone you're not; it's about fully embracing the incredible person you already are. It's about nurturing your self-worth and letting it shine through as you navigate the complex and beautiful landscape of motherhood.

So, as we delve into this chapter on boosting self-confidence, remember that the journey begins within. You have the power to be your own best cheerleader, to acknowledge your worth, and to cherish the connection you have with yourself. It's a journey that may have challenges, but it's one that holds the promise of profound self-discovery and unshakable self-confidence.

The Maternal Confidence Conundrum

Maternal self-confidence is a precious commodity, one that can be both fragile and resilient. Yet, it's a commodity that often faces a barrage of external and internal pressures. Society sends us messages about what a "perfect" mother should be, and we internalize these standards, often to our own detriment.

Parenting, while immensely rewarding, can also be incredibly stressful. The demands of caregiving, juggling work and home life, and trying to meet our own needs can feel overwhelming. This stress can chip away at our self-confidence, making us doubt our abilities and decisions.

When maternal self-confidence wanes and stress becomes overwhelming, many of us resort to coping mechanisms that provide temporary relief but do not address the underlying issues. Excessive phone use, alcohol consumption, and caffeine reliance may offer moments of escape, but they can also perpetuate feelings of guilt and inadequacy.

Meditation: Building Confidence and Self-Worth

Find a quiet space where you can sit comfortably. Close your eyes and take a few deep breaths, inhaling deeply through your nose and exhaling slowly through your mouth.

Find a comfortable and quiet space where you can sit or lie down. Close your eyes and take a few deep breaths, inhaling deeply through your nose and exhaling through your mouth. Let go of any tension in your body with each breath.

Let us begin by grounding: Imagine yourself standing in a beautiful, serene forest.

Feel the solid ground beneath your feet, connecting you to the Earth's energy.

As you stand here, envision your body bathed in a warm, golden light or self-worth and confidence.

You are enough, imperfections in all, you are enough.

Begin to reflect on your strengths as a mother.

Think about the challenges you've faced and the hurdles you've overcome.

Visualize these experiences as stepping stones, each one making you stronger and more resilient.

Acknowledge that you are not perfect, and that's perfectly okay.

Embrace your imperfections with love and compassion.

Imagine each imperfection as a unique facet of the beautiful gem that makes you who you are.

As you continue to breathe deeply, bring your attention to your heart center.

Visualize a warm, radiant light glowing within your heart.

This light represents self-love and self-acceptance. Feel it expanding with each breath, filling every corner of your being.

Picture yourself creating a protective bubble of energy around you.

This bubble represents your boundaries. It is strong and impenetrable, allowing only positive energy to enter. Know that it's okay to say "no" when necessary and to prioritize your well-being.

Imagine a support network of loved ones surrounding you.

They offer their encouragement, understanding, and love. You are not alone in your journey.

"I am worthy of love and respect." "I believe in my abilities as a mother."

"I embrace my imperfections with love and compassion."

"I set healthy boundaries to protect my well-being."

Visualize yourself radiating with confidence and self-worth.

Gently bring your awareness back to the room.

Wiggle your fingers and toes, and when you're ready, open your eyes.

Carry this sense of enhanced self-worth and confidence with you as you continue your journey of motherhood.

Affirmation

"I believe in myself and my abilities as a mother."

Feel the warmth of self-confidence and self-worth radiate from within. Know that you are enough, just as you are, and that your journey as a mother is uniquely yours.

As you continue to breathe deeply, visualize your self-confidence growing stronger, like a resilient tree with deep roots. You are capable, you are strong, and you are worthy of self-belief.

Reflection

Boosting self-confidence as a mother is a journey of self-discovery and self-compassion. Here are some thoughts to consider:

1. **Challenging Societal Standards:** Recognize that societal standards of motherhood are often unattainable and unrealistic. Embrace your unique path and choices as a mother.

2. **Self-Compassion:** Practice self-compassion by treating yourself with the same kindness and understanding you would offer to a dear friend.

3. **Seeking Support:** Reach out to friends, family, or a therapist when stress and self-doubt become overwhelming. Sharing your challenges can help lighten the emotional burden.

4. **Healthy Coping Strategies:** Explore healthier coping strategies that promote self-care and self-regulation. These may include mindfulness, exercise, journaling, or seeking professional help.

5. **Embrace Imperfection:** Remember that imperfection is part of the journey. It's through our challenges and mistakes that we grow, learn, and become stronger.

Boosting self-confidence as a mother is not about striving for perfection; it's about recognizing your inherent worth and believing in yourself. Many of us may feel very alone in the journey of motherhood, proving we have resilience that lies deeper than any strength known to us.

Companionship on this road is always appreciated, but the more isolated, know that there are other women shouldering these burdens alone too. May you meet and be company for one another.

CHAPTER

13

Chapter 13: Relaxation for Busy Moms

In the whirlwind of a busy working mom's life, finding moments to unwind can seem like an elusive luxury. The demands of balancing work, parenting, and household responsibilities can leave us feeling perpetually frazzled. But I'm here to tell you that these moments of relaxation are not a luxury; they are essential to maintaining emotional regulation. In this chapter, we'll explore quick relaxation techniques, affirming that you can find moments of relaxation even in your busiest days.

The Burnout Trap

In the hustle and bustle of modern life, especially here in America, it's all too easy to get swept up in the vortex of non-stop motion. Our culture glorifies busyness, celebrates constant connectivity, and seems to applaud those who perpetually keep moving. But let me tell you, I've been there. I've been caught in the whirlwind, and I've experienced the consequences of forgetting to step out of the overly busy pace.

The speed of life in our country can be breathtaking, but it can also leave us breathless in another way. The pressure to keep doing more, achieving more, and staying connected to everything and everyone can become all-consuming. We find ourselves tethered to our schedules, addicted to the constant stream of notifications on our devices, and trapped in a cycle of perpetual motion.

But here's the paradox: more isn't always better. In fact, sometimes, more can lead to less—less time for ourselves, less time for our loved ones, and ultimately, less of the peace and well-being we crave.

It's an easy trap to fall into. I've experienced moments of burnout that were entirely avoidable had I remembered to step back and take a breath. There's immense value in recognizing the signs of burnout: the exhaustion, the emotional depletion, the sense of being on a treadmill that never stops.

In this chapter, we're going to explore the importance of relaxation for busy moms. It's a reminder that finding moments to unwind, even in the midst of our hectic lives, isn't a luxury—it's a necessity. It's a lifeline that can help us avoid the burnout trap and maintain our emotional well-being.

So, as we dive into quick relaxation techniques and affirmations to nurture your self-care, remember that it's okay to step out of the never-ending motion, to pause in the whirlwind, and to reclaim moments of tranquility in the midst of life's speed.

It's a choice that can make all the difference in your journey as a busy working mom.

The Tug-of-War in Motherhood

Motherhood, especially in the realm of a busy working mom, often feels like a relentless tug-of-war. You're pulled in multiple directions, juggling the demands of your career, the needs of your children, and the responsibilities of daily life. It's a balancing act that can leave little room for self-care.

But here's the secret: relaxation doesn't always require a quiet retreat or a spa day (though those are lovely when you can manage them). Instead, it's about seizing the moments, even the briefest ones, to release the tension and recharge.

Quick Relaxation Techniques: Let's explore some quick relaxation techniques that you can weave into your busy day:

1. **1-Minute Breathing:** Take just one minute to focus on your breath. Inhale deeply for a count of four, hold for four, and exhale for four. Repeat a few times to reset your nervous system.
2. **The Power of Nature:** If you have even a moment to spare, step outside and connect with nature. Feel the sun on your face, take

in the scent of flowers, or simply gaze at the sky. Nature has a remarkable way of grounding and soothing.

3. **Partner Support:** Don't hesitate to tap out occasionally. Rely on your partner or a trusted friend or family member to take over for a short break. If you're on this journey alone, I encourage you to find some trusted childcare, such as a reliable babysitter! Whether it's a solo walk or time to enjoy a favorite book, this support system can provide essential moments of relaxation.

Meditation: Pausing to Take a Breath

Find a comfortable and quiet space where you can sit or lie down. Close your eyes and take a few deep breaths, inhaling deeply through your nose and exhaling through your mouth. Let go of any tension in your body with each breath.

Begin by focusing your attention on your body, realizing the tension that your body has collected throughout the day.

Fill your lungs with a deep breath, allowing air to fill your entire body. Hold this breath briefly for 5 seconds, then release, allowing your whole being to deflate like a balloon, sinking into a state of relaxation.

Imagine this wave of relaxation starting at the top of your head and slowly moving down through your body.

Feel this wave of relaxation as it softens and eases any areas of tension or stress.

As you continue to breathe deeply, imagine any stress or worries as heavy stones in a backpack. One by one, take these stones out of your backpack and set them down on the ground.

Feel the weight lifting from your shoulders with each stone you release. You may experience a physical relaxation in your shoulders as they drop, releasing tension.

Visualize a gentle stream of healing energy flowing through your body.

This energy is renewing and revitalizing. It washes away any lingering stress or fatigue, leaving you feeling refreshed and energized.

Now, you are ready to return to a balanced state, with which you will resume your day.

Imagine yourself standing on a balance beam, perfectly centered and steady.

This balance represents the equilibrium between your responsibilities and self-care.

You remember that it is always permissible to take time for yourself and find this balance.

Remind yourself that you have permission to care for your needs and seek balance whenever stress becomes pressing.

Conclude with one, final deep breath.

Gently bring your awareness back to the room. Wiggle your fingers and toes, and when you're ready, open your eyes.

Carry this sense of balance, relaxation, and renewal with you as you return to your daily responsibilities. Remember that taking moments for self-care is essential to being your best self as a mother and in all areas of your life.

Affirmation

"I find moments of relaxation even in my busiest days."

Visualize yourself incorporating these quick relaxation techniques into your daily routine.

See yourself taking those precious moments to unwind, to reset, and to nourish your well-being.

Reflection

Relaxation is not a luxury; it's a necessity for maintaining emotional regulation and finding balance in the chaos of motherhood. Here are some thoughts to consider:

1. **Seizing Transition Moments:** Identify transition moments in your day when you can incorporate quick relaxation techniques. It could be during your commute, a lunch break, or even while waiting to pick up your child.
2. **Partnering for Support**: Don't hesitate to ask for support from your partner or loved ones. They can help create the space you need to unwind and recharge.
3. **Redefining Self-Care:** Understand that self-care doesn't always require grand gestures. Even a few moments of intentional relaxation can have a profound impact on your well-being.
4. **Guilt-Free Relaxation:** Release any guilt associated with taking time for yourself. Remember that self-care is an investment in your ability to be present and nurturing for your family.
5. **Consistency:** Make relaxation a consistent part of your routine. Over time, these moments of self-care will become a lifeline in the busyness of your life.

As a busy working mom, you have a reservoir of inner strength, but it's crucial to remember that even the strongest need moments of relaxation and rejuvenation. By incorporating these quick relaxation techniques and affirming your commitment to self-care, you're taking vital steps toward maintaining emotional regulation and finding moments of peace within the whirlwind of your days.

CHAPTER 14

Chapter 14: Joy Through Difficult Moments

There's no denying it—motherhood is filled with difficult moments and seasons that can be overwhelming. I'll be the first to admit that I had a hard time enjoying those newborn days because of how overstimulating the entire experience was for me. It can feel trite to encourage my fellow mothers to find joy in their children, but sometimes it's something we take for granted.

You see, your little ones are not your friends. They are incredible, wonderful, miraculous little beings that you have the privilege and responsibility of raising. And that care burden, truthfully, can feel like a lot sometimes. Okay, let's be real—often, it feels like a lot. Very often. But here's the perspective I want to offer: finding joy in those simple moments of motherhood is not only essential for your mental health but also for your child's well-being.

Joy is a powerful remedy against disconnection and the challenges that come your way. It's not always easy to find, especially when stress and exhaustion threaten to push joy to the back of your mind. But let's cultivate a bank of joyful moments, a reserve to draw upon during those challenging times. For me, joy often arises from gratitude and awe. It's the recognition that these little people, these bundles of energy and curiosity, came from my body and are learning how to be in the world.

Cultivating Gratitude through Guided Meditation

Find a quiet and comfortable place to sit or lie down. Close your eyes and take a few deep breaths, inhaling deeply through your nose and exhaling through your mouth. Let go of any tension in your body with each breath.

Let's shift your attention to the present moment.

Bring to the forefront of your mind a recent challenging situation or moment in your life, perhaps related to motherhood.

Acknowledge the difficulty, but also recognize that within every challenge, there are moments of beauty and growth.

Now, bring to mind something or someone you're grateful for. It could be a loving relationship, a simple pleasure, or a beautiful memory.

Visualize this source of gratitude in your mind's eye: perhaps it's the connection with your children, achieving milestones in your life or career.

Notice the warm glow of joy it ignites in your heart and mind. Imagine tis warmth spreading from your heart to the rest of your body. This light represents the joy that comes from gratitude.

See it expanding with each breath, filling your entire being with a sense of joy, warmth, and appreciation.

Repeat this affirmation silently or out loud: "I choose to find joy in every moment, even in challenges." "I am grateful for the lessons and growth that come with each experience." "I embrace the beauty of life with an open heart and gratitude."

Carry this sense of joy and gratitude with you as you navigate the challenges of motherhood and life. By fostering gratitude, you can find moments of joy even in the most trying times, enriching your journey as a mother and a person.

Affirmation

"I find joy and gratitude in every moment with my children."

As you continue to breathe deeply, immerse yourself in the joy and wonder of your child. Feel your heart swell with love and appreciation for their presence in your life.

Reflection

Finding joy in motherhood is not about denying the challenges or the difficult moments; it's about shifting your focus to the moments of connection, the shared laughter, and the simple pleasures. Here are some thoughts to consider:

1. **The Power of Presence:** Joy often emerges when we are fully present with our children. Be in the moment, free from distractions, and savor the connection.
2. **Gratitude Practice:** Cultivate a gratitude practice in your daily life. Regularly reflect on the things you appreciate about your children and your journey together.
3. **Reconnecting with Wonder:** Embrace your child's sense of wonder and awe. Sometimes, by seeing the world through their eyes, we rediscover our own capacity for joy.
4. **Self-Compassion:** Remember that it's okay to have challenging moments and days. Self-compassion allows you to navigate these times with greater ease.
5. **Share Joy:** Encourage a culture of joy in your home. Celebrate small wins, create moments of laughter, and express your love openly.

Finding joy in motherhood is not about glossing over the tough parts; it's about celebrating the beauty, the connection, and the awe-inspiring journey of raising little humans. By nurturing moments of joy and gratitude, you're not only receiving benefit but also creating an environment where your children can flourish.

CHAPTER
15

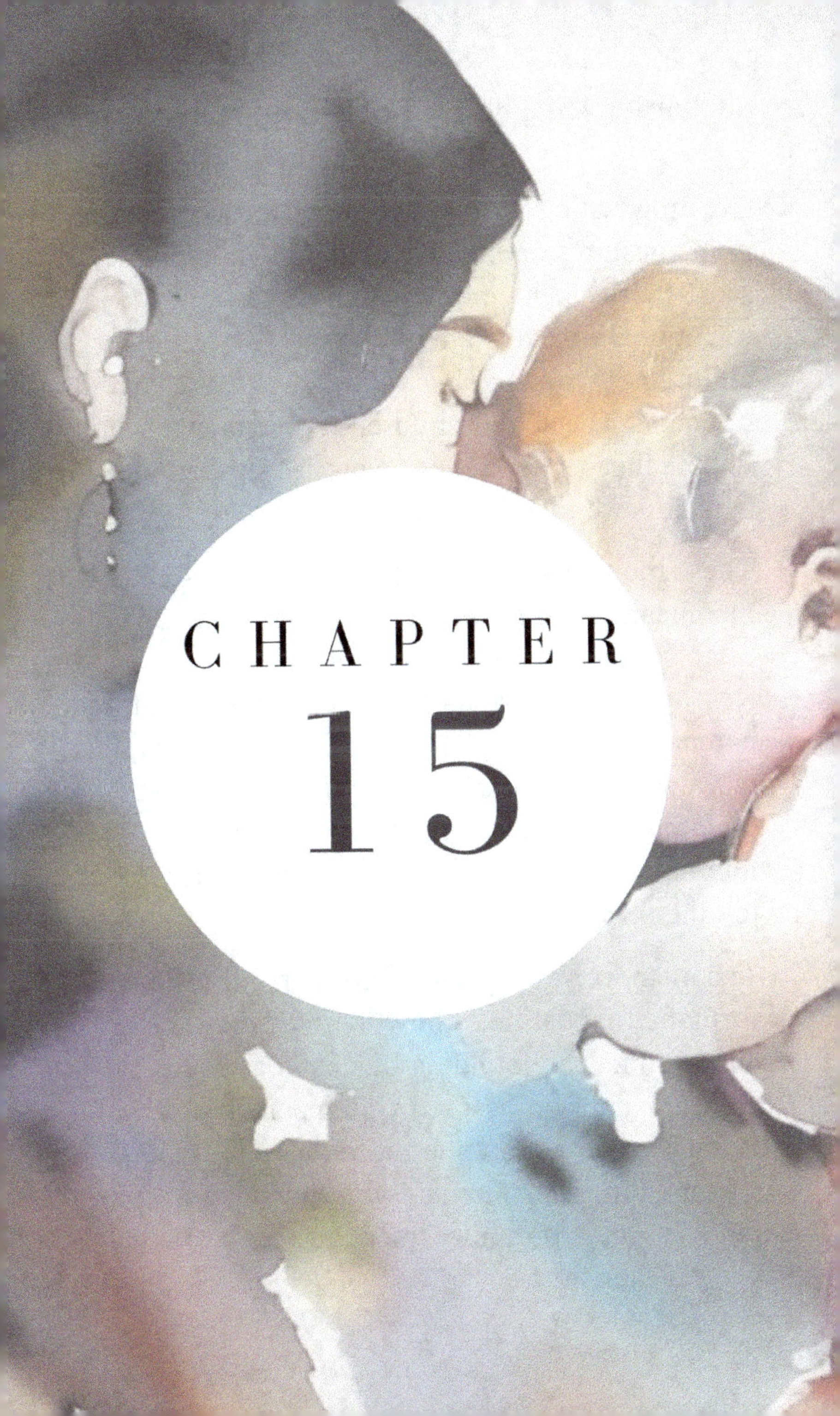

Chapter 15: The Gift of Lasting Memories

Creating lasting family memories doesn't require grand gestures or expensive outings. In fact, the most cherished memories often come from intentional time and attention that we give to our children. As we look back through life one day, the moments we and our children will remember most will be those small times where we support their formation of identity and personhood.

These moments foster a healthy sense of self, help them learn to attune to their own needs, and establish that they are loved and cared for. Research has shown us that intentional, nurturing parental attention reflects to a child their own sense of value: when we shower them with love, our children believe they are lovable, and they internalize a deep sense of self-worth because we tell them we love them.

The memories we aim to build with our little ones form the foundation of how they see themselves and become core building blocks of a secure, well-adjusted, and self-assured young person's identity. But it's not just about the future; it's about the present, too. Each moment you spend together as a family is an opportunity to create a memory that will be cherished.

My Aha Moment

As I delved into the concept of creating family memories, I couldn't help but reflect on my own love languages—those unique ways I both give and receive love. While I've always been aware of several love languages that resonate with me, one recently came to the forefront in a powerful way: gift-giving.

For as long as I can remember, I've taken immense joy in giving gifts to others. It's an expression of love and appreciation that fills me with happiness. But, there's a twist to this love language that I only recently discovered during a personal meditation. You see, I've often been teased by my husband about our cozy, small home, which occasionally feels cluttered.

In this moment of reflection, I realized that my love for gift-giving had sometimes taken on an unhealthy twist. It became a way for me to compensate for what I couldn't give in abundance—my time and presence. In those moments when life overwhelmed me, and I felt stretched thin, I found myself reaching for tangible items to fill the void. I gave gifts when I felt guilty about not being able to fully engage and give of myself.

But here's the revelation that hit me like a bolt of lightning: my children don't need more things. Their hearts aren't yearning for an abundance of toys or possessions. What they truly crave, what nourishes their souls, is the gift of my attuned presence in their lives. As their mother, my presence is the greatest gift I can offer them.

If you find yourself recognizing a similar pattern in your own journey—giving from a place of guilt or stretching yourself too thin to be fully present—I challenge you to sit with this realization a little deeper. Take a moment to re-parent your love language. Shift your focus from the tangible to the intangible, from material gifts to the priceless gift of being fully present.

I've learned that, as parents, our presence is the most valuable and cherished gift we can give our children. It's a gift that forms the foundation of their self-worth, their sense of love, and their cherished memories. So, let's challenge ourselves to nurture our relationships by being present, by creating moments of connection, and by savoring the beauty of our shared experiences as a family. This, I've come to realize, is the most enduring and meaningful way to create lasting family memories.

Affirmation

"I create cherished memories with my family."

Allow this affirmation to resonate within you, reinforcing your commitment to nurturing positive and loving memories with your own children.

Here is a further affirmation, affirming the value of presence over materialism:

"The most meaningful memories my children and I will make are the moments when I choose to be present to them, not the expensive experiences I could give them."

This affirmation underscores the importance of being fully present with our children and cherishing those moments of connection and love as the most valuable and lasting memories we can create together as a family.

Holding this affirmation in our minds and hearts, lets travel through a guided meditation to help us savor special moments with our children, despite all the chaos we may live through in the day to day.

Guided Meditation to Savor Special Moments

Let's embark on a guided meditation journey to savor special moments and reflect on the messages we remember from our parents, both the wounds and the affirmations:

Find a comfortable and quiet space where you won't be disturbed. Close your eyes and take a few deep breaths to center yourself.

Imagine a cherished memory from your own childhood—a moment when you felt loved, valued, and deeply connected to your parents or caregivers.

This memory might involve a simple act of kindness, a shared adventure, or a heartfelt conversation.

As you relive this memory, notice how it makes you feel. Pay attention to the warmth in your heart, the smile on your face, and the sense of security and love that washes over you.

Now, shift your focus to the present moment. Picture your own children—their smiles, laughter, and unique personalities.

Visualize a special moment you've shared with them recently or one you hope to create in the future.

Imagine yourself fully present in this moment with your children, just as your parents or caregivers were present for you. Feel the love and warmth between you and your little ones.

Reflect on the messages you remember from your parents—both the wounds you may still carry and the affirmations that have become a part of who you are.

Acknowledge the impact these messages have had on your own sense of self-worth and how they shape your interactions with your children.

Inhale deeply and say the following affirmation: "I will keep creating cherished memories with my family."

It is not necessary to fully heal from our own parenting wounds in order to be present to our own children and enjoy the small moments with them. They are unique and beautiful gifts in our lives, even if we struggle to be present to those small moments due to our own overwhelm. Be present to yourself in those moments. Breath, lean into the pain you are feeling, and allow it to coexist with the difference of your own children's experience now. Your job as a mother is to hold your childhood pain in tension with the experience you give to your children.

Reflection

Creating family memories is a profound and ongoing journey. Here are some thoughts to consider as you reflect on this meditation:

1. **The Power of Presence:** Being fully present with your children in the moment is the key to creating lasting memories. Let go of distractions and immerse yourself in the experience.
2. **Embracing Imperfection:** Remember that creating memories isn't about perfection. It's
3. about genuine connection, love, and authenticity.
4. **Healing the Past:** Reflect on the messages you received from your own parents. Identify any wounds or negative beliefs you may have inherited and work on healing and transforming them.
5. **Affirming Love:** Regularly express your love and affirmation to your children. Let them know how cherished and valued they are.
6. **Quality over Quantity:** It's not about the quantity of time but the quality of the moments you share. Simple, heartfelt interactions can create lasting memories.

Creating family memories is a gift that keeps on giving, both to your children and to yourself. Each cherished moment you create strengthens the bond between you and contributes to a sense of love, security, and self-worth that will shape your children's lives for years to come. So, let's continue this journey of creating beautiful memories with our families, one precious moment at a time.

CHAPTER

16

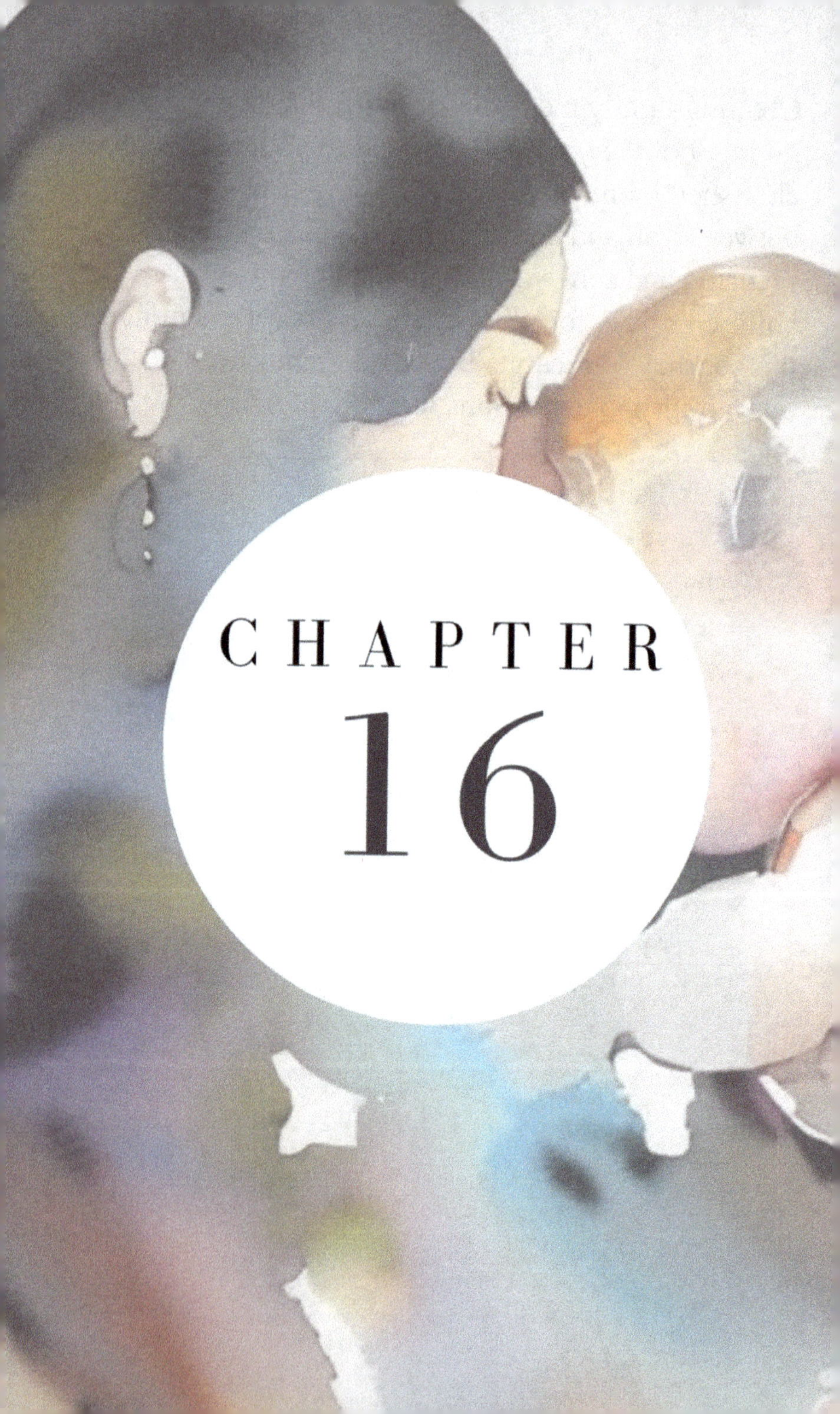

Chapter 16: Managing Overwhelm

As mothers, we often find ourselves on the front lines of life's chaos, juggling an array of responsibilities and navigating a complex emotional landscape. Overwhelm can strike at any time, leaving us feeling flooded and stretched thin. Some of us may wrestle with sensory overwhelm, while others grapple with intrusive thoughts or the stress associated with external pressures. For many, these challenges are compounded by the echoes of our own formative years.

It's crucial to understand that you don't have to have had a traumatizing or challenging childhood to struggle with overwhelm as a parent. However, if you did, these feelings can become more intense and complex. Neglect, abuse, or other adverse experiences from our past can resurface when we're faced with the absolute needs of our children—needs that rely on us for nourishment, safety, care, and modeling of healthy regulation skills.

Releasing Overwhelm through Guided Meditation

Let's embark on a guided meditation journey designed to help you cope with overwhelming moments, identify unmet needs from your own past, and learn to re-parent yourself while recognizing that it's okay to seek support when needed:

Find a quiet and comfortable space where you won't be disturbed.

Sit or lie down in a relaxed position, and take a few deep breaths to center yourself.

Close your eyes and imagine a moment when you felt completely overwhelmed as a parent.

Visualize the thoughts and emotions that swirled around you during that time.

Now, imagine yourself stepping out of that overwhelming moment, as if you're an observer looking in. Notice any patterns, triggers, or recurring thoughts that may surface.

As you observe, gently acknowledge any unmet needs from your own childhood that might be resurfacing in these overwhelming moments. These could be needs for validation, safety, or a sense of control.

Inhale deeply and say the following affirmation: "I am capable of handling any challenge that comes my way."

Affirmation

"I am capable of handling any challenge that comes my way."

Allow this affirmation to resonate within you, reminding yourself that you have the inner strength and resilience to face overwhelming moments.

Now, picture yourself as a child, with those unmet needs you've identified. Visualize yourself offering love, understanding, and care to that inner child. Imagine yourself meeting those unmet needs with compassion.

Return to the present moment, knowing that you carry this newfound awareness and compassion with you.

Reflection

Managing overwhelm is an ongoing journey, and it's important to normalize this feeling. Here are some thoughts to consider as you reflect on this meditation:

1. **Identifying Triggers:** Recognizing the triggers and patterns that lead to overwhelm is the first step in managing it. Pay attention to what sets you off and explore the underlying emotions.
2. **Re-parenting Yourself:** Just as we care for our children, we must learn to re-parent

ourselves by meeting our unmet needs with love and compassion.

3. **Seeking Support:** There's strength in seeking support when needed. Don't hesitate to lean on family, friends, partners, or therapists if you feel paralyzed in the face of your own needs.

4. **Balancing Self-Care:** Prioritize self-care as a means of replenishing your inner resources. Self-care isn't selfish; it's essential for your well-being.

5. **Understanding Your Past:** Reflect on your own childhood experiences and how they may influence your reactions to overwhelm. Understanding your past can help you navigate your present.

Managing overwhelm is a journey that requires self-awareness, self-compassion, and a willingness to seek support when necessary. Remember that you are capable of handling any challenge that comes your way. By acknowledging your own unmet needs, re-parenting yourself, and reaching out for support, you can find balance and resilience in the face of overwhelm.

I wanted to end this chapter on a more personal note, from my own parenting experience and reflection in therapy. Yes, we therapists see therapists too! I want to share a personal journey that has guided me toward a deeper understanding of managing my own sense of overwhelm as a mother. At times, I found myself repeating unhealthy patterns of interaction with my own children, especially during my lowest moments. For me, these moments often manifested as overstimulation, leading me to a place of yelling when I reached my own emotional breaking point.

I vividly recall moments when my children would shrink away, tears streaming down their faces, as my own emotions became so unmanageable that I couldn't care for them as they deserved. Witnessing their distress served as a wake-up call, a stark reminder that I needed support. My journey toward managing overwhelm isn't perfect, but it has come a long way. I've learned to monitor my own "overwhelm" meter, striving to manage my sensory needs proactively rather than letting them escalate suddenly.

When I find myself on the brink of meltdown, I've developed strategies to protect my children from the still-healing part of my inner child. One valuable tool has been taking space, when possible, and tapping out with my partner. This allows me to step away briefly and regain my composure. However, there are moments when leaving the overwhelming situation isn't feasible. For instance, when my older toddler is in the midst of a meltdown, refusing cooperation, and crying loudly, I've learned to practice grounded reflection. I sit down at her level, acknowledging how I see her expressing her feelings, recognizing that she too is overwhelmed.

Internally, I try to remind myself that her intense emotions aren't about me; she is struggling to cope. In those moments, my role is to provide her with a safe space to regulate her emotions. Sometimes, it's simply about holding her until she calms, offering gentle affirmations or the gift of quiet presence, and recharging myself when possible through sips of water or focused breathing exercises.

This practice isn't always easy, and I'm still learning. But it's about recognizing the cues that point to where re-parenting is still needed for my own inner child. It's about committing to response rooted in care and concern for that scared child within me. We're all on a journey, and healing takes time. By acknowledging our own struggles and taking intentional steps toward managing overwhelm, we can create a safer and more nurturing environment for our children as well as re-parenting and nurturing ourselves along the way.

CHAPTER

17

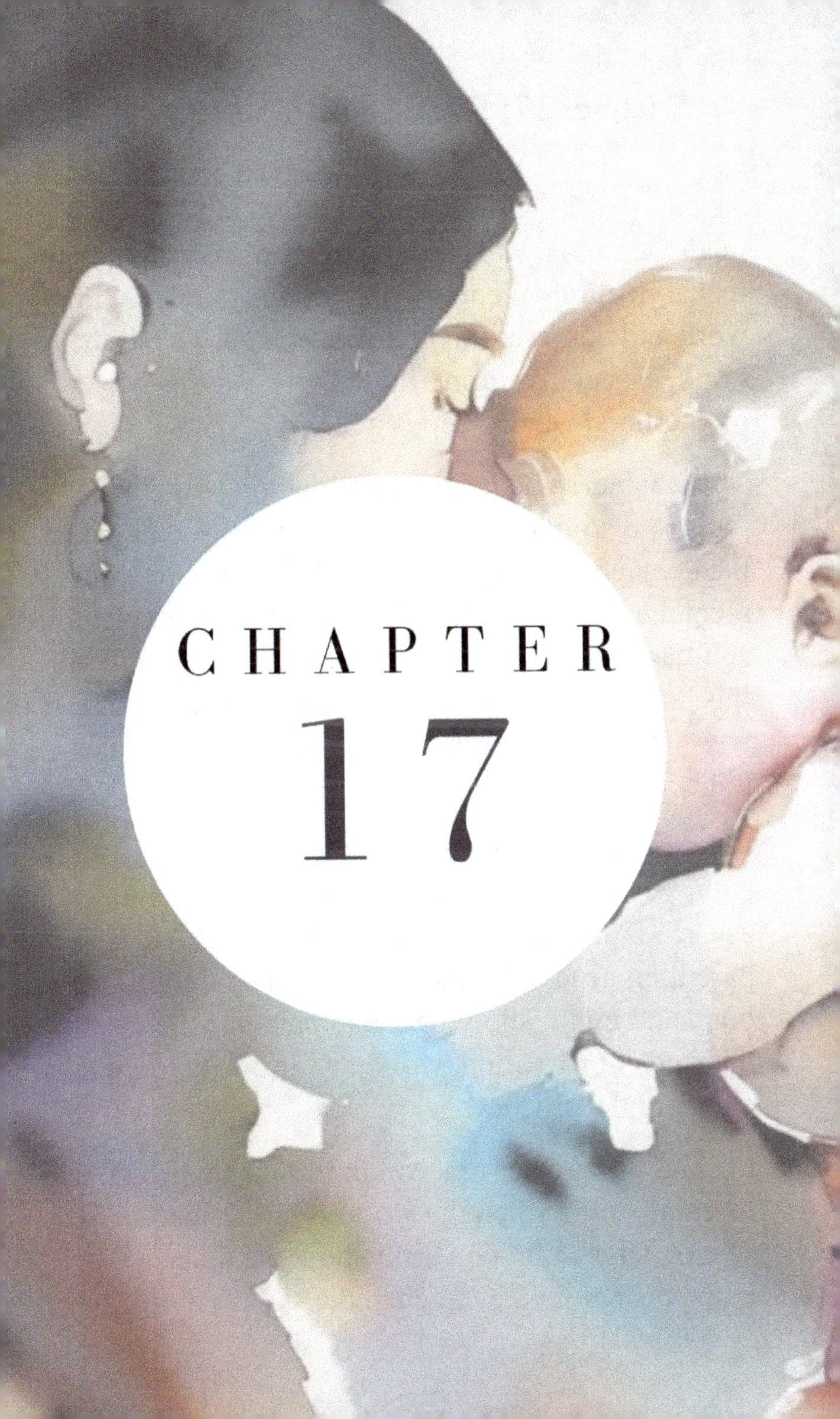

Chapter 17: Recharging Your Energy

As busy working mothers, we often find ourselves in a relentless cycle of caregiving, with little time to recharge our own energy. Parenting, coupled with work and daily responsibilities, can push us to the brink, especially during those early seasons of motherhood when sleep is a luxury.

This chapter is dedicated to providing you with tools to maintain your stamina and well-being when the demands of parenting are taking a toll on your mental and physical health. The key theme here is self-care because, as we've emphasized throughout this book, when our own needs are not being met, we cannot be as present and effective as we'd like to be for our children.

Let me start from a personal note: Recharging our energy is a deeply personal experience, as unique as each mother's journey and as varied as her re-parenting needs. For me, it's a ritual that aligns my body and mind, allowing me to navigate the demands of parenting, work, and life with more clarity and resilience.

I find my source of renewal in routine, in the early morning hours when the world is still asleep. There's something powerful about the quiet moments before dawn, when the sky is painted with the promise of a new day. It's a time when I can reliably step into my running shoes, embrace the pavement, and let the rhythm of my breath and footsteps ground me.

A morning run or other form of exercise has become my sanctuary—a sacred ritual that sharpens my body and mind. It fills me with a sense of strength and accomplishment, setting a tone for the day ahead. In those precious moments, I clear the clutter from my busy mind, allowing me to be more present for my family and the challenges of my work.

The beauty of recharging is that it's deeply personal. What rejuvenates one mother may not resonate with another. Some may find solace in a quiet cup of tea or a few pages of a good book. Others may seek refuge in a creative pursuit, a moment of meditation, or a heartfelt conversation with a friend.

As we explore the art of recharging in this chapter, remember that there's no one-size-fits-all approach. It's about discovering what replenishes your energy, aligns with your needs, and honors your journey of self-care and re-parenting. Whether you find solace in the tranquility of early mornings, the gentle embrace of evening yoga, or the simplicity of mindfulness, embrace the practices that fill your cup and restore your vitality.

The path to recharging is as unique as your fingerprint, and it's a journey well worth embarking on. It's not a luxury but a necessity—a means of preserving your well-being and nurturing the best version of yourself, not just for your own sake but for the precious ones who depend on your love and presence.

Recharging Your Inner Battery through Guided Meditation:

I've designed two options for guided meditation, each catering to specific moments when you need to recharge:

Option 1: Finding Balance at the End of a Long Day

Find a quiet, comfortable spot where you can sit or lie down without distractions. Take a few deep breaths to settle into the moment.

Close your eyes and visualize the end of a long, exhausting day.

See yourself setting aside the worries, stress, and responsibilities that have weighed on you.

Inhale deeply and exhale slowly, releasing the tension in your body with each breath. Let go of any worries or thoughts that may be crowding your mind.

Repeat the following affirmation: "I replenish my energy and vitality daily."

Affirmation

"I replenish my energy and vitality daily."

Imagine a serene place where you can sit and simply be. It could be a peaceful garden, a tranquil beach, or a cozy nook. Picture yourself there, feeling the warmth of the sun or the gentle breeze on your skin.

Sit in this mental sanctuary for a few moments, allowing yourself to fully relax and recharge.

Let's proceed with the second option for the guided meditation supporting our parental recharge throughout those hectic, busy days.

Option 2: Brief Recharge Throughout the Day

When you find yourself in need of a brief recharge during a busy day, take a moment to pause wherever you are.

It could be at your desk, in the car, or even in a quiet corner of your home.

Close your eyes and take a deep breath. Inhale deeply and exhale slowly.

Repeat a shortened version of the affirmation: "I take moments to replenish my energy."

Affirmation

"I take moments to replenish my energy."

Imagine a small, serene space where you can briefly escape the demands of the day. Visualize yourself there, even if only for a few minutes, feeling a sense of peace and calm.

As this chapter ends, reflect on the importance of self-care and re-parenting as essential components of recharging your energy. Just as we must seek to fill ourselves to avoid pouring from an empty cup, we also need to honor our own well-being to be the best versions of ourselves for our children.

Remember that self-care is a necessary act of self-preservation. By making time to recharge and meet your own needs, you not only enhance your own well-being but also create a more harmonious environment for your family. Recharging your energy isn't a luxury—it's an essential part of being the loving, present mother you aspire to be.

CHAPTER
18

Chapter 18: Resilience in Motherhood

Motherhood is a journey filled with challenges, tests, and moments that push us to our limits. We've explored the impact of our early childhood experiences and how they shape our paths as mothers. Now, we delve into the powerful concept of resilience—the inner strength and adaptability that enable us to thrive in the face of adversity.

Throughout this book, we've acknowledged that our mother figures, well-intentioned as they may be, can both nurture our sense of self and leave us with deep childhood wounds. It's essential to recognize that we all do our best with the tools we've been given, and sometimes, our mother figures' own unmet needs may have contributed to our own struggles.

Resilience in motherhood is about understanding that parenting will test us in ways we never imagined. From the sleepless nights to financial pressures, medical anxieties, concerns about our children's development, and the social pressures they face—it's an endless list of challenges. And yet, a parent's job never ends; we can't simply quit or take a day off. It's an ongoing, transformative journey where we learn and grow together with our children.

Building Resilience and Inner Strength through Guided Meditation:

In this guided meditation, we invite you to lean deeply into the lessons you've learned and set intentions to keep growing and staying open. Embrace the growth mindset that allows you to learn with and from your experiences, adapting to the ever-changing landscape of motherhood.

Find a quiet, comfortable space where you can sit or lie down without distractions. Take a few deep breaths to center yourself in the present moment.

Close your eyes and imagine yourself standing on the shores of a vast, serene lake.

This lake represents your journey as a mother—calm and still on the surface, but deep and full of experiences beneath.

Visualize the water, representing your inner resilience. Notice how it reflects the world around it, mirroring your environment and the challenges you face.

Take a moment to acknowledge the strengths you possess as a mother. Think about the times you've shown patience, kindness, and love to your children.

Visualize these moments as shining stars above the lake's surface, illuminating the path ahead.

Now, shift your focus to the challenges you've encountered on this journey.

These challenges are like ripples on the lake's surface, sometimes causing turbulence.

Acknowledge them without judgment, recognizing that they are a natural part of your experience.

As you continue to breathe deeply, think about the driving forces—the emotions—that prompt your responses to your children.

These emotions are like currents in the lake, shaping your reactions and interactions.

Observe the emotions you feel most frequently in your role as a mother.

Are they love, joy, frustration, or exhaustion? Let these emotions surface in your mind's eye, allowing them to be present.

Repeat the following affirmation: "I am resilient and adaptable as a mother."

Affirmation

"I am resilient and adaptable as a mother."

Imagine yourself embracing both the strengths and challenges, as well as the driving forces of your emotions. See them all as interconnected, like elements of nature working in harmony.

As we reflect on the concept of resilience in motherhood, I'm reminded of the incredible strength that resides within each of us. It's a strength born from the understanding that we are not perfect, and we will make mistakes. It's a strength rooted in the knowledge that our journey as mothers is a continuous process of learning and evolving.

Our children are our greatest teachers, and they offer us daily opportunities to grow in compassion, patience, and resilience. When we recognize and acknowledge our own moments of vulnerability and imperfection, we model for them the beauty of self-acceptance and the power of growth.

Remember, resilience is not about being unbreakable; it's about being adaptable and open to change. It's about embracing the challenges of motherhood with courage and the willingness to learn from each experience. You are stronger and more resilient than you may realize, and your journey as a mother is a testament to your incredible capacity for growth and transformation.

CHAPTER
19

Chapter 19: Practicing Healthy Boundaries

Setting boundaries in motherhood is a vital practice that extends from our earlier discussions about external pressures, internal influences, and the journey of re-parenting ourselves. It's an integral part of developing our capacity to be present and balanced parents.

Drawing boundaries within a family can be one of the most challenging aspects of motherhood. We may fear guilt, judgment, or even the possibility of straining relationships. However, it's essential to remember that boundaries are not about creating distance but about nurturing healthy connections.

Boundaries are like the protective fence around a garden. They allow your family to flourish, grow, and thrive in an environment that prioritizes well-being. They enable you to attune to your inner child's unmet needs and create a safe space for your family to develop and thrive.

As mothers, we have a profound responsibility to protect and prioritize our children's well-being. This includes setting boundaries that support their growth and development. Each family is unique, and it's crucial to consider your own family unit's needs and your own well-being when establishing these boundaries.

Boundaries are a way of honoring your family's journey, your own growth, and your commitment to creating a loving and nurturing environment. They serve as a reminder that you are the guardian of your family's well-being and happiness, and your ability to set boundaries is an act of love and protection.

Meditation: Establishing Healthy Boundaries

Find a quiet, comfortable space where you can sit or lie down without distractions. Take a few deep breaths to center yourself in the present moment.

As you continue to breathe deeply, bring your awareness to your own boundaries.

Picture them as a delicate web that surrounds you, protecting your sense of self. Notice how your boundaries have evolved over the years, influenced by your childhood experiences and life's challenges.

Now, gently explore any wounds or triggers from your past that have contributed to the development of your boundaries.

These could be moments of hurt, neglect, or any other experiences that left an imprint on you. Without judgment, simply acknowledge them and observe how they have shaped your boundaries.

Place your hand over your heart and take a moment to offer yourself compassion.

Recognize that you are doing your best to heal and protect yourself, just as any loving parent would for their child. Embrace yourself with kindness and understanding.

Imagine a soft, golden light surrounding you, representing healthy and well-defined boundaries.

Picture this light growing stronger and more radiant with each breath. As it expands, it creates a safe and nurturing space within and around you.

Repeat this affirmation silently or out loud: "I honor my boundaries, knowing they are born from a place of love and self-protection."

"I allow myself to set healthy boundaries with compassion and understanding."

"I am creating a safe and nurturing space for myself and my family."

Take a few more deep breaths, feeling the strength of your boundaries and the compassion you've offered yourself.

When you're ready, gently open your eyes and return to the present moment.

Affirmation

"I set boundaries that support my well-being and my family's."

Recognize that, as mothers, it is our responsibility to protect our children and set priorities for their well-being.

While some families may expect unlimited access to their children, it's essential to consider your own family unit's needs and your own well-being when agreeing to family and external engagements.

Visualize yourself walking along the garden's boundary, reinforcing it with love and intention. Feel the strength and clarity that comes from setting healthy boundaries that honor your family's needs.

As you return to the present moment, carry with you the understanding that boundaries are not meant to separate families but to provide healthy paths of connection. They are a way of ensuring that your family thrives, protected by the love and care you provide.

I understand that drawing boundaries with a wounded inner child can be challenging, because that younger self wants to act in a way that that child feels will fulfill an unmet need. Our wounded inner children developed out of some boundary that did not exist in a healthy way while we were growing up, and it is essential to recognize the unhealthy pattern of interaction to which we have become accustomed.

It is on us as the parent to learn healthy patterns of relationship to teach out children. It is our responsibility as the parent to meet not only their physical needs, but their emotional needs. Through setting boundaries for our family, we protect our ability to meet the needs of our children.

A Guide to Setting Boundaries

Boundaries are an essential part of maintaining a healthy family environment. They serve as the protective fence around your family's well-being, ensuring that your loved ones thrive. Here are some ways to set and maintain boundaries effectively:

1. **Open Communication:** Invite family members and loved ones to be a part of the boundary-setting process. Explain why certain boundaries are essential for your family's well-being, and encourage them to share their perspectives as well.
2. **Be Clear and Specific:** Clearly define the boundaries you want to establish. Vague boundaries can lead to misunderstandings

and conflicts. Ensure that everyone understands what is expected and why.

3. **Consistency:** Consistency is key to successful boundary setting. Be firm in maintaining the established boundaries, and ensure that they are consistently applied. This helps create a sense of predictability and safety for your family.

4. **Prioritize Self-Care:** Setting boundaries also means prioritizing your own well-being. Recognize that self-care is not selfish but necessary for you to be the best parent you can be. Communicate this need to your family and enlist their support.

5. **Flexible Boundaries:** While boundaries are important, they should also be flexible when necessary. Be open to adjusting boundaries as your family's needs change over time. Flexibility can help maintain a healthy balance.

6. **Respect Others' Boundaries:** Just as you set boundaries for your family, respect the boundaries of others. Show understanding and empathy toward the boundaries that your extended family members or friends may need to set for their own well-being.

7. **Seek Professional Guidance:** If you are struggling to set boundaries or experiencing challenges with family members respecting

them, consider seeking the guidance of a therapist or counselor. They can provide valuable insights and strategies.

8. **Create a Support System:** Lean on your partner, close friends, or support groups for help in maintaining boundaries. Having a support system can make it easier to navigate challenging situations.

Remember that boundaries are not meant to limit love or create distance but to foster a healthy and nurturing environment for your family. They are a way of prioritizing your family's well-being and allowing everyone to grow and thrive in a space of love and respect.

As mothers, asserting our desires and intentions, especially when it comes to setting boundaries for our families, can be an internal struggle. We often grapple with questions like, "Am I being too demanding?" or "Will this cause conflict?" These internal battles are a testament to the depth of our love and care for our precious littles.

Our children are our world, and we want nothing but the best for them. Yet, sometimes, the best thing we can do is set boundaries that protect their well-being. It's not about being rigid or controlling; it's about creating a safe and nurturing space for them to grow and flourish.

So, as you embark on this journey of boundary setting, remember that it's a reflection of your deep love and commitment to your family. It's a way of saying, "I want the best for you, and I'm willing to navigate these challenges to ensure your happiness and safety." You are not alone in this struggle. Many mothers, including myself, have faced the same internal battles. But it's through these challenges that we learn and grow, both as individuals and as parents.

CHAPTER 20

Chapter 20: Celebrating Our Transformation in Motherhood

Motherhood is a remarkable journey, filled with challenges, triumphs, and endless opportunities for growth and healing. In this final chapter, we celebrate not only our roles as mothers but also the nurturing maternal figures who have guided us on this profound path.

Meditation:
Celebrating Your Role as a Mother

Find a quiet, comfortable space where you can sit or lie down. Close your eyes and take a few deep breaths to center yourself in the present moment.

As you settle into this moment, take a few deep breaths and reflect on the journey of motherhood. Picture yourself standing at the threshold of this incredible adventure.

Notice the path before you, winding through moments of joy, challenge, and growth.

Imagine walking along this path, and as you do, you may encounter moments or memories that trigger emotions from your own childhood.

These may be moments of longing, pain, or unresolved emotions. With compassion, allow these memories to surface and acknowledge the impact they've had on your journey.

As you continue on your path, visualize a younger version of yourself standing nearby. This is your inner child, who may still carry wounds from the past.

Approach her with love and care, just as you would comfort your own child. Offer her words of reassurance, hugs, and the understanding she needed but may not have received in the past.

As you walk further, you'll come across moments of pure joy and connection with your children.

Relive these moments in your mind, savoring the laughter, the hugs, and the simple pleasures of motherhood. Let these moments fill your heart with warmth and gratitude.

As you continue, you may encounter challenges and struggles you've faced as a mother.

These moments have also contributed to your growth and strength. Acknowledge the lessons you've learned and the resilience you've developed along the way.

Repeat the following affirmations silently or out loud: "I honor my journey as a mother, embracing both the joys and challenges." "I nurture my inner child, offering her the love and understanding she deserves." "I celebrate the incredible growth and strength I've gained through motherhood."

Take a few more deep breaths, appreciating the journey you've walked as a mother. When you're ready, gently open your eyes and return to the present moment.

Remember that motherhood is a unique and ever-evolving journey, filled with both light and shadow.

By acknowledging and celebrating this journey, you are honoring your own growth and the love you provide to your children.

Affirmation

" I celebrate the incredible journey of motherhood, through its hardships and its joys."

Recognize that celebrating motherhood is not about perfection but about embracing the love, dedication, and resilience that define your role as a mother.

As mothers, we often find ourselves navigating uncharted waters, facing uncertainties, and questioning our abilities. But it's in these moments of vulnerability that we discover our true strength and capacity for love.

I've learned that celebrating motherhood means celebrating ourselves—our imperfections, our growth, and our unwavering commitment to our families. It means honoring the nurturing figures who have walked this path before us, offering guidance and wisdom. Each day, we have the opportunity to nurture, protect, and shape the lives of our precious children. We may stumble, and we may doubt, but we keep moving forward because our love is boundless.

Throughout this book, we have explored the profound journey of motherhood and the invaluable role you play in your child's life. Here are the key points we have discussed:

1. **The Power of Loving Attention**: We've learned that the attention and care you provide as a mother are more impactful in nurturing confident and resilient children than any material gift. Your love and presence are the greatest gifts you can give.
2. **Healing Through Intentional Work:** We've recognized that many of our struggles as mothers can be traced back to the insecurities left by incomplete parenting in our own younger selves. However, through intentional re-parenting and self-reflection, we have the power to heal and grow.
3. **The Art of Repair:** We've emphasized that it's okay to stumble and make mistakes in our parenting journey. What truly matters is our

willingness to repair and reconnect with our children when we do. These moments of repair can be transformative and strengthen our bonds.

4. **The Practice of Presence:** We've celebrated the importance of practicing presence with our children. Being fully engaged and attuned to their needs not only nurtures their well-being but also makes us more resilient mothers, capable of navigating the challenges of motherhood with grace.

As you continue on your journey of motherhood, remember that you are capable, resilient, and filled with love. Embrace the lessons learned, the growth experienced, and the joy found in every moment with your precious children. You are making a lasting impact on their lives, one filled with love, care, and the celebration of the incredible journey of motherhood. Let us embrace the journey, knowing that it's not about reaching a destination but about savoring the beauty of every moment.

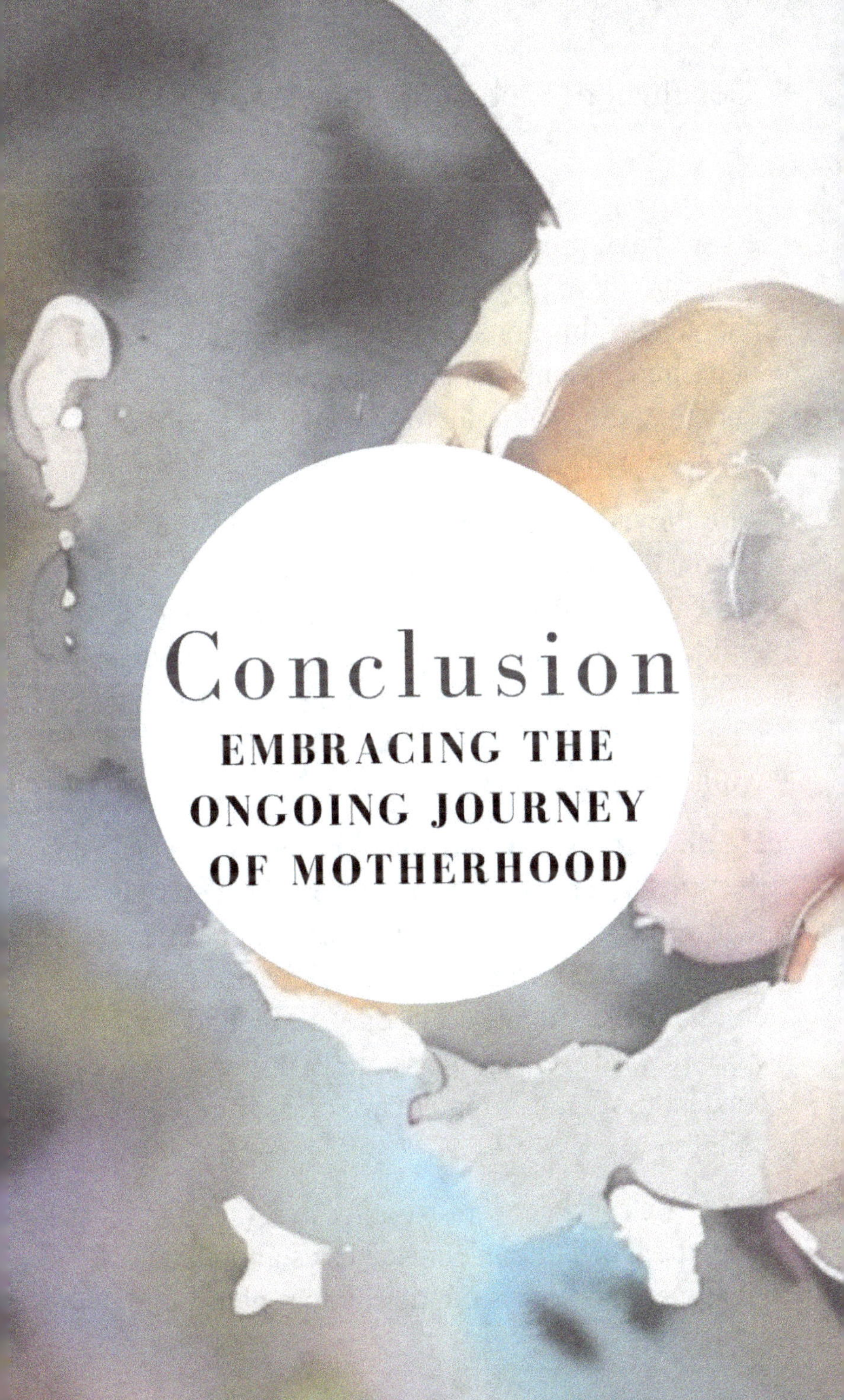
Conclusion
EMBRACING THE
ONGOING JOURNEY
OF MOTHERHOOD

Conclusion: Embracing the Ongoing Journey of Motherhood

As we have progressed together on the transformative journey of motherhood through the chapters of this book, I want to share some personal notes and lessons that have shaped my understanding of motherhood, and I hope they resonate with you too.

The Power of Presence: One of the most profound lessons I've learned as a mother is that being present is a gift we can give to ourselves and our children every day. It's not about always having the right answers or doing everything perfectly; it's about showing up with an open heart and a willingness to connect.

Healing and Re-parenting: Through my work as a therapist and my own experiences, I've come to realize that our journey as mothers often reflects the healing and re-parenting we need for our own inner child. It's okay to acknowledge our wounds and work towards self-compassion. In doing so, we create a more nurturing environment for our children.

Never be too Proud to Repair: I've stumbled, lost my patience, and made mistakes as a mother. But what matters most is our ability to repair the ruptures in our relationships with our children. These moments of repair can be powerful catalysts for growth, resilience, and deeper connections.

Boundaries to Encourage Health and Wholeness: Drawing boundaries can be challenging, especially when faced with external pressures and expectations. But I've found that setting healthy boundaries is an act of self-love and protection for our families. It's about creating space for growth, intimacy, and well-being.

Celebrate Your Journey of Growth as a Mother

Motherhood is a journey filled with highs and lows, joys and challenges. It's about celebrating the small victories, finding joy in everyday moments, and recognizing the incredible growth and transformation that both we and our children experience. As you continue your own unique journey of motherhood, keep these personal lessons in mind:

1. **Embrace Imperfection:** I've learned that perfection is an illusion. Embrace your imperfections, and let them be a source of growth and connection. Vulnerability is a pathway to authenticity.
2. **Cultivate Resilience:** Motherhood can be tough, but you are tougher. Embrace challenges as opportunities for resilience and personal

growth. You are capable of handling whatever comes your way.

3. **Prioritize Self-Care:** Self-care is not selfish; it's a necessity. Prioritize your well-being, recharge your energy, and remember that taking care of yourself enables you to care for your family more effectively.

4. **Practice Presence:** Every moment with your children is an opportunity for connection. Put away distractions, look into their eyes, and savor the beauty of the present. These moments are the building blocks of lasting bonds.

5. **Seek Support:** You don't have to navigate this journey alone. Seek support when needed, whether from friends, family, or professionals. Strength comes from recognizing when you need help.

6. **Celebrate the Journey:** Finally, celebrate the incredible journey of motherhood. Embrace the ups and downs, the messy moments, and the milestones. Your love and presence are shaping the future.

Thank you for allowing me to be a part of your journey. Embrace the journey, keep learning, and cherish the beauty of motherhood in all its imperfect, magnificent glory. The impact you make on your children's lives is immeasurable.

About the Author

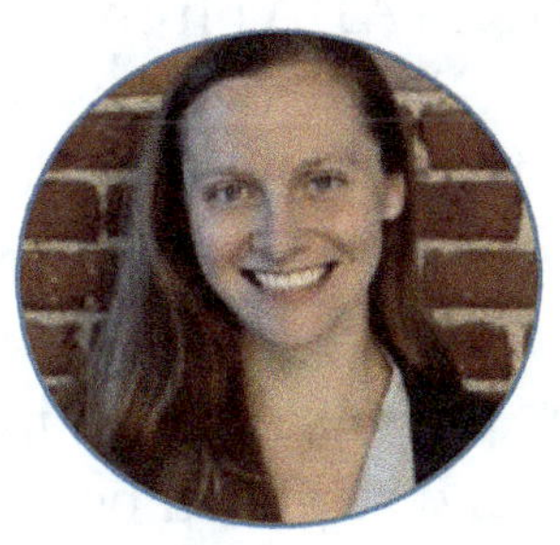

Hannah Mecaskey Conley is the mother of two wonderful balls of toddler energy, married to a fabulous partner and co-parent Joe, living in the Greater Boston Area. Hannah has been running a private practice alongside her public health career, Innovative Social Solutions, LLC., for the past 3 years. This book is the product of Hannah's own journey of self-discovery and re-parenting, finding her path relevant to many other young mothers and parents seeking to shape an emotionally intelligent childhood for their children. A consistent theme that has resonated in Hannah's clinical work with parents since 2016 is the need for parents to model and embody emotional regulation for their children in order for those children to be capable of managing big feelings.

Hannah is an experienced clinician and public health leader, working in the behavioral health field for over 14 years. Her clinical social work was obtained in 2016 from Case Western Reserve in Cleveland, Ohio. Hannah simultaneously completed her Master of Education in Applied Behavioral Analysis (ABA) from University of Cincinnati in 2016. These degrees provided Hannah with a career pivot from her first educational direction, when she studied philosophy and theology in Berkeley, CA from 2008 until 2013, obtaining Masters of Arts degrees in both disciplines. Hannah completed her educational journey in October 2020, just before the birth of her first child, completing a Doctorate in Behavioral Health Management at Arizona State University (2020).

While her academic journey may be complete, or at least paused at this time, Hannah welcomes those who find meaning in managing their own feelings to join her in her journey.

Hannah has launched her business website at: www.innovativesocialsolutionsllc.com

Join Hannah on Instagram at:

@MillennialMommingIt
@InnovatingSocially

www.ingramcontent.com/pod-product-compliance
Lightning Source LLC
Chambersburg PA
CBHW050815260726
48660CB00004B/1447